CLINICAL
PEDIATRIC
DERMATOLOGY

9.00

369 0240369

This book is due for return on or before the last date shown below.

CLINICAL
PEDIATRIC
DERMATOLOGY

Jayakar Thomas

MD DD MNAMS PhD FAAD

FRCP (Edin, Glasgow, London, Ireland), FRCPCH (London)

Professor and Head

Department of Skin and STD

Sree Balaji Medical College

Chennai, Tamil Nadu, India

Parimalam Kumar

MD DD Dip NB

Professor and Head

Department of Dermatology

Thanjavur Medical College

Thanjavur, Tamil Nadu, India

JAYPEE BROTHERS MEDICAL PUBLISHERS (P) LTD

New Delhi • London • Philadelphia • Panama

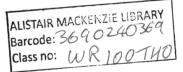

Jaypee Brothers Medical Publishers (P) Ltd

Headquarters

Jaypee Brothers Medical Publishers (P) Ltd
4838/24, Ansari Road, Daryaganj
New Delhi 110 002, India
Phone: +91-11-43574357
Fax: +91-11-43574314
Email: jaypee@jaypeebrothers.com

Overseas Offices

J.P. Medical Ltd
83 Victoria Street, London
SW1H 0HW (UK)
Phone: +44-2031708910
Fax: +02-03-0086180
Email: info@jpmedpub.com

Jaypee Brothers Medical Publishers Ltd
The Bourse
111 South Independence Mall East
Suite 835, Philadelphia, PA 19106, USA
Phone: + 267-519-9789
Email: joe.rusko@jaypeebrothers.com

Jaypee Brothers Medical Publishers (P) Ltd
Shorakhute, Kathmandu
Nepal
Phone: +00977-9841528578
Email: jaypee.nepal@gmail.com

Jaypee-Highlights Medical Publishers Inc.
City of Knowledge, Bld. 237, Clayton
Panama City, Panama
Phone: +507-301-0496
Fax: +507-301-0499
Email: cservice@jphmedical.com

Jaypee Brothers Medical Publishers (P) Ltd
17/1-B Babar Road, Block-B, Shaymali
Mohammadpur, Dhaka-1207
Bangladesh
Mobile: +08801912003485
Email: jaypeedhaka@gmail.com

Website: www.jaypeebrothers.com
Website: www.jaypeedigital.com

© 2013, Jaypee Brothers Medical Publishers

Inquiries for bulk sales may be solicited at: jaypee@jaypeebrothers.com

This book has been published in good faith that the contents provided by the authors contained herein are original, and is intended for educational purposes only. While every effort is made to ensure accuracy of information, the publisher and the authors specifically disclaim any damage, liability, or loss incurred, directly or indirectly, from the use or application of any of the contents of this work. If not specifically stated, all figures and tables are courtesy of the authors. Where appropriate, the readers should consult with a specialist or contact the manufacturer of the drug or device.

Clinical Pediatric Dermatology

First Edition: **2013**

ISBN 978-93-5090-455-8

Printed at: Ajanta Offset & Packagings Ltd., New Delhi

Dedicated to

The many devoted practitioners who provide skin health to children, to our committed teachers of Dermatology, and most of all to our beloved spouses for their care love and affection without which this humble piece of work would not have been a reality.

PREFACE

"Knowledge, if not shared is of no use at all".

Over the years, pediatric dermatology has emerged as a vital field of medical practice, yet with paucity of sufficient printed teaching material.

This book *Clinical Pediatric Dermatology (CPD)* is intended to serve three sections of physicians—pediatricians, dermatologists, and general practitioners.

An introductory chapter on examination of a child with a dermatologic problem is included to highlight the need for an astute clinical examination which brings the physician closer to the correct diagnosis. We have reiterated this by using flow charts.

Although basic in its early chapters, the *CPD* is definitely not elementary in the sense of 'putting' it to practice.

To write an introductory text alone would leave many readers with only a taste of the conceptual elements but no guidance for venturing into genuine practical applications.

Indeed, given the conceptual simplicity of this *CPD*'s approach, it is only hoped that the publication of this book will enhance the spread of ideas that are currently trickling through the scientific literature.

We wish you happy and fruitful reading!

Jayakar Thomas
Parimalam Kumar

CONTENTS

Structure and Functions of Skin

Dermatological problems are seen by pediatricians everyday and comprise of around one quarter of a busy outpatient clinic. Most children and adolescents present with skin disorders can be easily diagnosed and treated. This chapter will present a brief account of some such skin conditions.

STRUCTURE AND FUNCTIONS OF SKIN

The integument or skin covers the entire external surface of the human body and is the principal site of interaction with the surrounding world. It serves as a protective barrier preventing internal tissues from exposure to trauma, ultraviolet radiation, extreme temperature, toxins, and bacteria. Other important functions include sensory perception, immunologic surveillance, thermoregulation, and control of insensible fluid loss.

The skin consists of 2 mutually dependent layers, the epidermis and dermis, that rest on a fatty subcutaneous layer, the subcutis. The epidermis is derived primarily from surface ectoderm but is colonized by pigment-containing melanocytes of neural crest origin, antigen-processing Langerhans' cells of bone marrow origin, and pressure-sensing Merkel cells also of neural crest origin. The dermis is derived primarily from mesoderm and contains collagen, elastic fibers, blood vessels, sensory structures, and fibroblasts. During the fourth week of embryologic development, the single cell thick ectoderm and underlying mesoderm begin to proliferate and differentiate. The specialized structures formed by the skin, including teeth, hair, hair follicles, fingernails, toenails, sebaceous glands, sweat glands, and apocrine glands also begin to appear at approximately this period in development. Teeth, hair, and hair follicles are formed by the epidermis and dermis, while the epidermis alone forms fingernails and toenails. Hair follicles, sebaceous glands, sweat glands, apocrine glands, and mammary glands

Structure of skin

➤ **Layers**
   Epidermis
   Keratinocytes, Melanocytes, Langerhans, Merkel cells
   Dermis
   Cell—fibroblast, mast cells,
   Fibers—Collagen, reticular, elastic
   Structures—Blood vessel, lymphatics, nerve
   Substance—Mucopolysaccharides, chondroitin sulfates, glycoproteins
   Subcutis
➤ **Appendages of skin**
   Glandular—apocrine eccrine, sebaceous
   Nongladular—hair, nail
➤ **Layers of the epidermis**
   Stratum germinatum
   Stratum spinosum
   Stratum granulosum
   Stratum lucidum (palm and sole)
   Stratum corneum
➤ **Layers of the dermis**
   Superficial papillary dermis
   Deeper reticular dermis
➤ **Layers of dermoepidermal junction**
   Lamina lucida
   Lamina densa

are considered epidermal glands or epidermal appendages, because they develop as downgrowths or diverticula of the epidermis into the dermis. The definitive multilayered skin is present at birth, but skin is a dynamic organ that undergoes continuous change throughout life as outer layers are shed and replaced by inner layers. Skin also varies in thickness among anatomic location, sex and age of the individual. This varying thickness primarily represents a difference in dermal thickness, as epidermal thickness is rather constant throughout life and from one anatomic location to another. Skin is thickest on the palms and soles of the feet (1.5 mm), while it is thinnest on the eyelids and in the postauricular region (0.05 mm). Children have relatively thin skin, which progressively thickens until the fourth or fifth decade of life after which it begins to thin. This thinning is also primarily a dermal change, with loss of elastic fibers, epithelial appendages, and ground substance. The epidermis contains no blood vessels and is entirely dependent on the underlying dermis for nutrient delivery and waste disposal via diffusion through the dermoepidermal junction. The epidermis is a stratified squamous epithelium consisting primarily of keratinocytes in progressive stages of differentiation from deeper to more superficial layers. The named layers of the epidermis include the stratum germinativum, stratum spinosum, stratum granulosum, and stratum corneum. The stratum germinativum or basal layer is immediately superficial to the dermoepidermal junction. This single cell layer of keratinocytes is attached to the basement membrane via hemidesmosomes.

As keratinocytes divide and differentiate, they move from this deeper layer to the more superficial layers. Once they reach the stratum corneum, they are fully differentiated keratinocytes devoid of nuclei and are subsequently shed in the process of epidermal turnover. Cells of the stratum corneum are the largest and most abundant of the epidermis. This layer ranges in thickness from 15 to 100 or more cells depending on anatomic location and is the primary protective barrier from the external environment. Melanocytes, derived from neural crest cells, primarily function to produce a pigment, melanin, that absorbs radiant energy from the sun and protects the skin from the harmful effects of ultraviolet radiation. Melanin accumulates in organelles termed melanosomes that are incorporated into dendrites anchoring the melanosome to the surrounding keratinocytes. Ultimately, the melanosomes are transferred to the adjacent keratinocytes where they remain as granules. Melanocytes are found in the basal layer of the epidermis as well as in hair follicles, the retina, uveal tract, and leptomeninges. These cells are the sites of origin of melanoma. In areas exposed to the sun, the ratio of melanocytes to keratinocytes is approximately 1:4. In areas not exposed to solar radiation, the ratio may be as small as 1:30. Absolute numbers of melanosomes are the same among the both sexes and various races. Differing pigmentation among individuals is related to the size of melanosomes and their interspacing rather than cell number. Sun exposure, melanocyte-stimulating hormone (MSH), adrenocorticotrophic hormone (ACTH), estrogens, and progesterones stimulate melanin production. With aging, a decline is observed in the number of melanocytes populating the skin of an individual. Since these cells are of neural crest origin, they have no capability to reproduce. Langerhans cells originate from the bone marrow and are found in the basal, spinous, and granular layers of the epidermis. They serve as antigen-presenting cells. They are capable of ingesting foreign antigens, processing them into small peptide fragments, binding them with major histocompatibility complexes, and subsequently presenting them to lymphocytes for activation of the immune system. An example of activation of this component of the immune system is contact hypersensitivity. Merkel cells, also derived from neural crest cells, are found on the volar aspect of digits, in nailbeds, on the genitalia, and in other areas of the skin. These cells are specialized in the perception of light touch.

The primary function of the dermis is to sustain and support the epidermis. The dermis is a more complex structure and is composed of 2 layers, the more superficial papillary dermis and the deeper reticular dermis. The papillary dermis is thinner, consisting of loose connective tissue containing capillaries, elastic fibers, reticular fibers, and some collagens. The reticular dermis consists of a thicker layer of dense connective tissue containing larger blood vessels, closely interlaced elastic fibers, and coarse bundles of collagen fibers arranged in layers parallel to the surface. The reticular layer also contains fibroblasts, mast cells, nerve endings, lymphatics, and epidermal appendages. Surrounding the components of the dermis is the gel-like ground substance, composed of mucopolysaccharides (primarily hyaluronic acid), chondroitin sulfates, and glycoproteins. The deep surface of the dermis is highly irregular and borders the subcutaneous layer, the panniculus adiposus, which additionally cushions the skin. The fibroblast is the major cell type of the dermis. These cells produce and secrete procollagen and elastic fibers. Procollagen is terminally cleaved by proteolytic enzymes into collagen that aggregates and becomes cross-linked. These tightly cross-linked collagen fibers provide tensile strength and resistance to shear and other mechanical forces. Elastic fibers constitute less than 1% of the weight of the dermis, but they play an enormous functional role by resisting deformational forces and returning the skin to its resting shape. The dermoepidermal junction is an undulating basement membrane that adheres the epidermis to the dermis. It is composed of 2 layers, the lamina lucida and lamina densa. The lamina lucida is thinner and lies directly beneath the basal layer of epidermal keratinocytes. The thicker lamina densa is in direct contact with the underlying dermis. These structures are the target of immunologic injury in diseases such as bullous pemphigoid and epidermolysis bullosa. Epidermal appendages are intradermal epithelial structures lined with epithelial cells with the potential for division and differentiation. These are important as a source of epithelial cells,

Functions of skin

- Protective barrier
- Sensory perception
- Immunologic surveillance
- Thermoregulation
- Control of insensible fluid loss
- Sociosexual communication

Epidermal appendages

➤ **Sebaceous glands**
  Holocrine glands,
  Found over the entire surface of the body except palms, soles, dorsum of feet
  Largest and concentrated in the face and scalp
  Produce and secrete sebum, (triglycerides and fatty acid breakdown products, wax esters, squalene, cholesterol esters, and cholesterol)
➤ **Eccrine glands**
  Found over entire surface of the body except lips, external ear canal, and labia minora
  Most concentrated in the palms and soles
➤ **Apocrine glands**
  Concentrated in axillae anogenital regions
➤ **Hair follicles**
  Found over the entire surface of body except soles, palms, glans penis, clitoris, labia minora, mucocutaneous junction and portions of the fingers and toes
➤ **Specialized structures**
  Merkel cells, Meissner corpuscles—detect light touch
  Pacini corpuscles—pressure
  Krause bulbs—cold
  Ruffini corpuscles—t heat
  Naked nerve endings—Pain transmission

which accomplish re-epithelialization should the overlying epidermis be removed or destroyed in situations such as partial thickness burns, abrasions, or split-thickness skin graft harvesting. Epidermal appendages include sebaceous glands, sweat glands, apocrine glands and hair follicles. They often are found deep within the dermis, and in the face may even lie in the subcutaneous fat beneath the dermis. This accounts for the remarkable ability of the face to re-epithelialize even the deepest cutaneous wounds. Sebaceous glands, or holocrine glands, are found over the entire surface of the body except the palms, soles, and dorsum of the feet. They are largest and most concentrated in the face and scalp where they are the sites of origin of acne. The normal function of sebaceous glands is to produce and

secrete sebum, a group of complex oils including triglycerides and fatty acid breakdown products, wax esters, squalene, cholesterol esters, and cholesterol. Sebum lubricates the skin to protect against friction and makes it more impervious to moisture. It also has antimicrobial properties. Sweat glands, or eccrine glands, are found over the entire surface of the body except the lips, external ear canal, and labia minora. They are most concentrated in the palms and soles of the feet. Each gland consists of a coiled secretory intradermal portion that connects to the epidermis via a relatively straight distal duct. The normal function of the sweat gland is to produce sweat, which cools the body by evaporation. The thermoregulatory center in the hypothalamus controls sweat gland activity through sympathetic nerve fibers that innervate the sweat glands. Sweat excretion is triggered when core body temperature reaches or exceeds a set point. Apocrine glands are similar in structure but not identical to eccrine glands. They are concentrated in the axillae and anogenital regions. They probably serve a vestigial sexual function, because they produce odor and do not function prior to puberty. Hair follicles are complex structures formed by the epidermis and dermis. They are found over the entire surface of the body except the soles, palms, glans penis, clitoris, labia minora, mucocutaneous junction and portions of the fingers and toes. Sebaceous glands often open into the hair follicle rather than directly onto the skin surface, and the entire complex is termed the pilosebaceous unit. The base of the hair follicle, or hair bulb, lies deep within the dermis and in the face may actually lie in the subcutaneous fat. A band of smooth muscle, the arrector pili, connects the deep portion of the follicle to the superficial dermis. Contraction of this muscle, under control of the sympathetic nervous system, causes the follicle to assume a more vertical orientation. Hair growth exhibits a cyclical pattern. The anagen phase is the growth phase, whereas the telogen phase is the resting state. The transition between anagen and telogen is termed the catagen phase. Phases vary in length according to anatomic location, and the length of the anagen phase is proportional to the length of the hair produced. At any one time at an anatomic location, follicles are found in all 3 phases of hair growth.

Cutaneous vessels ultimately arise from underlying named source vessels. Each source vessel supplies a 3-dimensional vascular territory from bone to skin termed an angiosome. Adjacent angiosomes have vascular connections via reduced caliber (choke) vessels or similar caliber (true) anastomotic vessels. The cutaneous vessels originate either directly from the source arteries (septocutaneous or fasciocutaneous perforators) or as terminal branches of muscular vessels (musculocutaneous perforators). They emerge from the deep fascia in the vicinity of the intermuscular or intramuscular septa or near tendons and travel toward the skin, where they form extensive subdermal and dermal plexuses. The dermis contains horizontally arranged superficial and deep plexuses, which are interconnected via communicating vessels oriented perpendicular to the skin surface. Cutaneous vessels ultimately anastomose with other cutaneous vessels to form a continuous vascular network within the skin. Clinically, this extensive horizontal network of vessels allows for random skin flap survival. In addition to the skin's natural heat conductivity and loss of heat from the evaporation of sweat, convection from cutaneous vessels is a vital component of thermoregulation. Cutaneous blood flow is 10–20 times that required for essential oxygenation and metabolism, and large amounts of heat can be exchanged through

the regulation of cutaneous blood flow. The thermoregulatory center in the hypothalamus controls vasoconstriction and vasodilatation of cutaneous vessels through the sympathetic nervous system. Skin lymphatics parallel the blood supply and function to conserve plasma proteins and scavenge foreign material, antigenic substances, and bacteria. Blind-ended lymphatic capillaries arise within the interstitial spaces of the dermal papillae. They course through the deep dermal and subdermal plexuses and numerous filtering lymph nodes on their way to join the venous circulation near the subclavian vein-internal jugular vein junction bilaterally. Sensory perception is critically important in the avoidance of pressure, mechanical or traumatic forces, and extremes of temperature. Numerous specialized structures are present in the skin to detect various stimuli. Merkel cells of the epidermis detect light touch. Meissner corpuscles also detect light touch. These are found in the dermal papillae and are most concentrated in the fingertips. Pacini corpuscles are found deep within the dermis or even in the subcutaneous tissue. These structures are specialized to detect pressure. Pain is transmitted through naked nerve endings located in the basal layer of the epidermis. Krause bulbs detect cold, whereas Ruffini corpuscles detect heat. Heat, cold, and proprioception also are located in the superficial dermis. Cutaneous nerves follow the route of blood vessels to the skin. The area supplied by a single spinal nerve, or single segment of the spinal cord, is termed a dermatome. Adjacent dermatomes may overlap considerably, of importance to note when performing field blocks with local anesthesia.

Approach to History Taking and Clinical Examination in Children with Dermatologic Problems

INTRODUCTION

Any small blemish on the skin causes great concern to the parents and children. The adolescents feel that they are being looked at with social dislike. That is why 'dysmorphophobia' a relatively new terminology has come into very common use, particularly when considering the demands among adolescent patients with dermatological problems. This is essentially because adolescents are establishing a sense of autonomy by scrutinizing, modifying, or rejecting their parents' values and instead comparing and identifying with the standards of their peer group. The 'internal struggle' between being dependent and independent, at the same time, results invariably in non-compliance of treatment. For the above reasons, as in any other specialty, history taking, clinical examination, laboratory examination, and treatment carry a specific adolescent-friendly pattern. The physician must describe the pros and cons of treatment

and explicitly leave the choice and responsibility of implementation to the adolescent.

This chapter covers the following:
1. Approach to history taking.
2. Approach to physical examination.
3. Basic relevant investigations.

APPROACH TO HISTORY TAKING

History varies from case to case, so one should be prepared for the same and finer details of history elicited. The following are guidelines towards a comprehensive approach.

Recording of identification information should be supplemented with details like
- Place of dwelling for endemic disease like varicella
- Close living in hostel as in scabies, pediculoses, viral, and fungal diseases
- Occupation as in oil folliculitis and oil acne.

History taking must include:

- Chief complaints
- Present history
- Past history
- Personal history
- Family history
- Treatment history
- Psychological assessment of the patient and parents.

Chief Complaint/s

The complaint/s may be present since birth, e.g. Nevoid conditions like hemangiomas, epidermal nevus or can be of later onset.

If later in onset, note down the complaint/s in chronological order with duration, e.g.

1. Red lesions for 6 months.
2. Sudden increase in redness and scaling almost all over body for 1 week, as in psoriatic erythroderma.

Present History

This includes the following:

History detailing complaint/s

- Nature of symptoms, like itching, burning, photosensitivity, pain, etc.
- Evolution and progress of the disease—duration and location of symptoms, constant or periodic and localized or generalized. Record the evolution like a vesicle changing into a bulla, which easily ruptures to leave large erosions, e.g. pemphigus
- Alterations by therapy and seasonal variation. History related to systemic association, e.g. fever and joint pains as in systemic lupus. History to rule out *close differentials,* e.g. presence of psoriatic plaque to differentiate psoriatic erythroderma from drug-induced erythroderma. History to *initiate treatment,* e.g. to rule out hepatic problem, immunodeficiency, and hematological abnormality, if methotrexate is planned.

History *to rule out complications and for follow-up,* e.g. diarrhea to rule out dermatogenic enteropathy as a complication of erythroderma; development of joint pains as in systemic lupus erythematosus.

Past History

This includes history detailing similar illness, related illness, other illness, whether hospitalization was required and details of treatment.

Personal History

Meticulous eliciting of personal history, as below, gives clues towards diagnosis and etiology:

- Use of cosmetics (allergic contact dermatitis), garments (textile dermatitis)
- Dietary habit e.g. wheat exacerbates dermatitis herpetiformis
- Habit of smoking, alcohol (can worsen Psoriasis)
- Recreational history, e.g. swimming followed by sun burns
- Travel history, e.g. leishmaniasis. Atopy, diabetes, hypertension, thyroid disease
- History of exposure to the risk of sexually transmitted infections and also drug abuse
- History of transfusion
- Menstrual history: Flare during or before menstruation as in autoimmune progesterone dermatitis/urticaria.

Family History

It must include history of similar illness, related illness, other illness, whether hospitalization was required and details of treatment in the family members.

Treatment History

Record in detail the dose, duration, and effects of all drugs used by the patients, which includes:

- Topical and systemic treatment for the current illness, to choose further therapy
- Short-term treatment (last 3 weeks) for adverse cutaneous drug reactions
- Long-term treatment, e.g. clofazimine treatment for leprosy for brownish black discoloration of skin
- Treatment for other disease, e.g. steroids for bronchial asthma resulting in acneiform eruptions/striae.

Psychological Assessment of the Patient

Depressed patient can have dermatitis artefacta.

Assessment of the Parents

Overzealous parents may over-treat their child.

▌APPROACH TO PHYSICAL EXAMINATION

Examination must include the following:
- General examination
- Systemic examinations
- Dermatological examination.

General and Systemic Examinations

General examination and systemic examinations should be done as for other systems.

The need for the above is exemplified below, as a primary dermatological problem may be a reflection of systemic diseases and vice *versa*.
- Respiratory system, e.g. reduced chest expansion as in progressive systemic sclerosis
- Cardiovascular system, e.g. pulmonary stenosis as in LEOPARD syndrome
- Abdomen, e.g. hepatomegaly as in mastocytosis and storage disorders
- Central nervous system, e.g. sensory impairment as in trophic ulcers.

One has to bear in mind that diseases like Stevens-Johnson syndrome, toxic epidermal necrolysis (TEN), drug reactions, erythroderma, etc. should be considered as 'dermatological emergencies'. Adequate caution is required while examining these patients.

Dermatological Examination

Undress patients to the extent needed. Examine under adequate illumination. While examining, one has to remember the following:
- Requisites for a routine dermatological examination
- Identify primary and secondary lesions
- Distribution and configuration
- Examination of hair, nails, mucosae, peripheral nerves.

Requisites for a Routine Dermatological Examination

- Torch
- Hand lens × 10 magnification
- Glass slide
- Blunt needle
- Wisp of cotton
- Knee hammer
- Inch tape
- Test tubes with hot and cold water.

Dermatological examination includes examination of the entire skin, including scalp, palms and soles, mucosae, hair nail and peripheral nerves, if Hansen's disease is suspected.

The signs of the skin diseases are called lesions, and it is usual to call them "the Alphabet". By being able to recognize the letters, you can put them together and form words and sentences that have meaning. These lesions or the "Alphabet" are classified into primary and secondary. When a lesion develops without a preceding manifest skin change, it is primary. But when a lesion changes in character, even by its natural evolution in time, it becomes secondary.

Identify Primary and Secondary Lesions
Primary lesions
Macule: Circumscribed area of altered color without textural change less than 1 cm in size.

Flow chart 2.1: Identification of disease through pigmented macule/patch

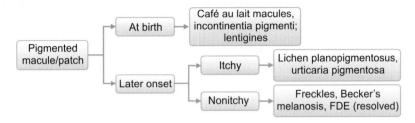

Flow chart 2.2: Identification of disease through hypopigmented patch

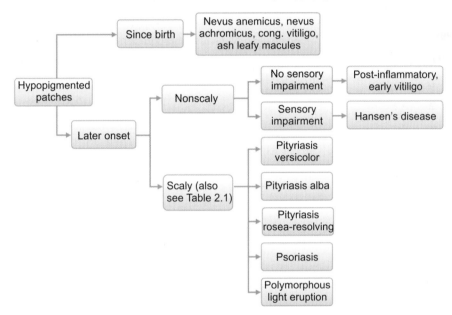

Examples:
Pigmented—café au lait spot (Flow chart 2.1)
Hypopigmented—ash leafy macule
Depigmented—vitiligo
Erythematous—pityriasis rosea (PR)
Scaly—pityriasis versicolor

Patch: Circumscribed area of altered color without textural change more than 1 cm in size.

Examples:
Pigmented—fixed drug eruption (FDE), resolving
Hypopigmented—Hansen's disease (Flow chart 2.2 and also Table 2.1)
Depigmented—vitiligo
Erythematous—nevus flammeus
Annular—tinea corporis
Scaly—psoriasis

Papule: Circumscribed solid elevation of the skin less than 1 cm size.

Examples:
Skin-colored—syringoma (Flow chart 2.3)
Pigmented—angiofibroma
Erythematous—insect bite allergy
Hemorrhagic—meningococcemia
Violaceous—lichen planus (Flow chart 2.4)
Yellow—xanthoma
Scaly—psoriasis
Verrucous—wart
Dome-shaped—molluscum contagiosum
With a punctum—molluscum contagiosum
Pedunculated—neurofibroma
Grouped—lichen nitidus

Table 2.1: Symptoms in various hypopigmented skin diseases					
	Pityriasis versicolor	Pityriasis alba	Pityriasis rosea	Psoriasis	Polymorphous light eruption
Border	Pencil-drawn	Ill-defined	Well-defined	Well-defined	Irregular
Scaling	Fine, uniform	Coarse	Peripheral collarette	Silvery	Scales may or may not be present
Sign	Fingernail sign			Auspitz sign	Dyschromatosis
Others	Asymptomatic	Recurs and reappears at different sites	Herald patch followed by profusion of lesions	Nail/scalp involvement	Photosensitivity

Flow chart 2.3: Identification of disease through skin-colored papule

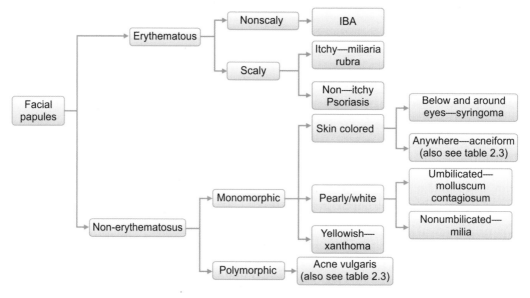

Flow chart 2.4: Identification of disease through pigmented papule

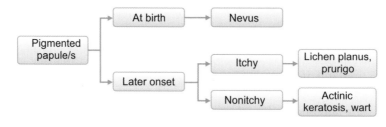

Grouped accuminate and follicular—Pityriasis rubra pilaris

Plaque: Circumscribed alteration in the skin either raised above or sunk below.

Examples:
Atrophic—discoid lupus erythematosus (DLE)
Hypertrophic—keloid
Verrucous—tuberculosis verrucosa cutis (Flow chart 2.5)

Flow chart 2.5: Identification of disease through verrucous plaque

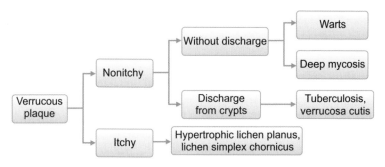

Vesicle: Circumscribed visible collection of clear fluid in the skin less than 1 cm.

Examples:
Discrete—miliaria crystalina
Grouped—herpes simplex
    On an erythematous base and segmental—Herpes zoster

Bulla: Circumscribed visible collection of clear fluid in the skin more than 1 cm (Table 2.2).

Examples:
Flaccid—pemphigus
Tense—bullous pemphigoid

Pustule: Circumscribed visible collection of pus in the shin (Flow chart 2.6).

Examples:
Nonfollicular—pustular psoriasis
Follicular—folliculitis
Lake of pus—pustular psoriasis

Cyst: Collection of fluid or solid matter contained within a wall in the skin.

Examples:
Follicular—epidermal cyst
Nonfollicular—dermoid cyst

Nodule: Raised solid lesion more than 1 cm in the epidermis, dermis or subcutis.

Example:
Erythema nodosum

	Pemphigus	Erythema multiforme (drug-induced)	Pemphigoid	Dermatitis herpetiformis
Itching	(–)	+	+/–	++
Mucosal involvement	+	+	(–)	(–)
Base	Normal skin	Normal/ erythematous	Erythematous/ edematous	Normal
Nature of bulla	Flaccid	Tense	Tense	Grouped vesicles
Shape of bulla	Irregular	Round	Dome-shaped	(–)
Sign/feature	Nikolsky, Asboe-Hansen signs	Target lesions, iris lesions	Nil	Nil
Post-inflammatory change	Pigmentation/ acanthoma	Milia	Hypopigmentation	Excoriations
Others	Paronychia	Scarring—mucosal		Enteropathy

Table 2.2: Signs and symptoms of diseases due to full a formation

Flow chart 2.6: Identification of diseases through primary pustular eruption

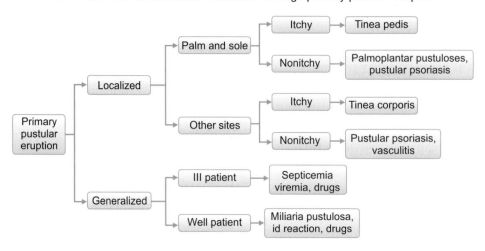

Ulcer: Discontinuity in the epidermal surface with loss of dermal tissue.

Example:
Tropical ulcer

Tumor: Solid mass of skin or subcutaneous tissue larger than 1 cm (does not always mean the lesion is neoplasm).

Example:
Neurofibroma

Wheal: Transient, erythematous dermal edema.

Example:
Urticaria

Burrow: S-shaped tunnel in the upper epidermis.

Example:
Scabies

Comedone: Solid elevation with plug of keratin and sebum within the pilosebaceous orifice (Table 2.3).

Example:
Acne vulgaris

Telangiectasia: End vessel dilatation.

Example:
Poikiloderma

Purpura: Red unblanchable spot due to bleed into the skin. Ecchymosis refers to larger lesions.

Examples:
Palpable—Henoch Schönlein purpura
Nonpalpable—Idiopathic thrombocytopenic purpura

Erythema: Red blanchable spot due to increased blood flow into the skin.

Example:
Urticaria

Target lesion: Annular patch or plaque with central vesicle or cyanosis, with halo of erythema.

Example:
Erythema multiforme (EMF)

Secondary lesions

Scale: Visible shedding of stratum corneum (Flow chart 2.7).

Examples:
Fine branny scale—pityriasis versicolor
Silvery scale—psoriasis

Table 2.3: Characteristic features of acneiform eruption and acne

	Acneiform eruption	Acne
Age	Any age	Adolescent
Sex	M = F	M > F
Onset	Sudden	Gradual
History of drug intake	Yes	No
Site	Any site	Seborrheic areas
Distribution	Trunk > Face	Face > Trunk
Lesions	Monomorphic	Polymorphic
Comedones	Absent	Always present
Cysts	Not seen (excepting in cyclosporine-induced)	Seen in severe forms
Scarring	No	Yes

Flow chart 2.7: Identification of disease through scaly plaque

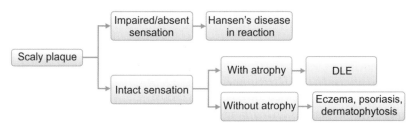

Peripheral collarette—Pityriasis rosea
Adherent scale—Discoid lupus erythematosus
Asbestos like—Tinea amiantacea

Crust: A dried collection of blood, serum, or pus and cell debris.

Examples:
Honey colored—Impetigo
Hemorrhagic—EMF

Erosion: Superficial loss of surface epithelium with intact dermis.

Example:
Intertrigo

Excoriation: Loss of surface epithelium by scratching or rubbing, exposing the dermis.

Example:
Acne excorie

Fissure: Linear cleavage of the surface epithelium/skin (Flow chart 2.8).

Example:
Skin—Fissured feet
Mucocutaneous junction—candidal balanitis

Scar: Fibrous replacement of lost dermal connective tissue.

Examples:
Atrophic—DLE
Hypertrophic—Acne
Ice pick—Acne
Cribriform—Pyoderma gangrenosum
Tissue paper—Epidermolysis bullosa
Cigarette paper—Ehlers-Danlos syndrome

Eschar: Hard darkened plaque covering an ulcer implying extensive tissue necrosis, infarct or gangrene.

Flow chart 2.8: Identification of disease through fissured feet

Example:
Echthyma

Lichenification: Plaque with increased thickening, pigmentation and accentuated skin markings.

Example:
Lichen simplex chronicus

Atrophy: Loss of or thinning of epidermis, dermis or subcutis. More than one portion can be involved.

Examples:
Epidermal—steroid induced
Dermal—lichen scleroses et atrophicus
Subcutis—atrophoderma
Perifollicular—acne

Sclerosis: Area of indurated skin that is bound down and difficult to be pinched.

Examples:
Localized—morphea
Generalized—scleroderma

Pits: Shallow depression in the epidermis.

Example:
Pitted keratolysis

Ulcer: Discontinuity in the epidermal surface with loss of dermal tissue (Table 2.4).

Example:
Tropical ulcer

Distribution, Pattern, and Configuration

Not only is the appearance of lesions important, but the distribution, pattern, and configuration on the skin is as well. Also take note of the surface changes, feel, signs and special features of each lesion as given below.

Distribution
Sun exposed area—PLE
Exposed area (uncovered by cloth)—papular urticaria/IBH
Seborrheic area—seborrheic dermatitis
Curve of Hebra—scabies
Scalp, elbows, knees, lumbosacral—psoriasis
Bathing trunk/suit—pityriasis rosea
Butterfly area—SLE
Follicular—LPP, phrynoderma,
Dermatomal—herpes zoster

Pattern and configuration
Annular: Annular lesions are seen in a ring shape mostly with central clearing (Flow chart 2.9).

Table 2.4: Signs and symptoms in various ulcer types

	Arterial	Venous	Neuropathic	Tropical
Pain	Yes	No, but itchy	No	Yes
Other history	Intermittent claudication	Edema leg	Depending on cause	Constitutional symptoms
Site	Distal limb	Above medial malleolus	Pressure points	Shin
Size	Small	Large, encircling the leg	Small to medium	Small to medium
Type	Punched out	Shallow to deep	Punched out	Shallow to deep
Floor	Necrotic eschar	Yellow slough	Granulation tissue	Unhealthy granulation tissue
Margin	Well-defined	Irregular	Well-defined	Well-defined
Discharge	No	Yes, if infected	Yes, if infected	Yes, dribbling down the leg
Surrounding skin	Cold	Pigmented and later indurated	Anesthetic, callosity present	Normal
Other findings	Feeble peripheral pulse	Varicose veins	Peripheral nerve thickening, loss of deep tendon reflex in diabetics	Signs of malnutrition

Flow chart 2.9: Identification of disease through annular lesions

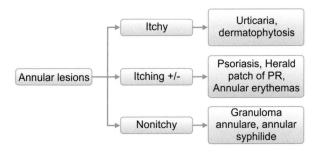

Examples:
Itchy Tinea corporis
Nonitchy Granuloma annulare

Discrete: Discrete lesions tend to remain separate. This is a helpful descriptive term but has little specific diagnostic significance.

Example:
Varicella

Clustered: Clustered lesions are those that are grouped together (Flow chart 2.10).

Examples:
Vesicle – herpes simplex
Papule – insect bites

Confluent: Confluent lesions tend to run together.

Examples:
Confluent and reticulated papillomatosis

Dermatomal, zosteriform: Dermatomal, zosteriform lesions follow a dermatome and are mostly unilateral.

Flow chart 10: Identification of disease through grouped lesions

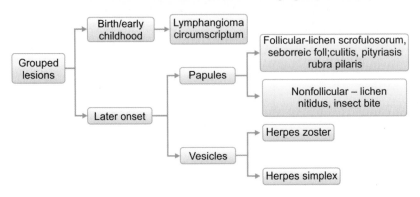

Example:
Herpes zoster

Follicular: Lesions are folliculocentric, helpful to determine if lesions specifically involve the hair follicle (Flow chart 2.11).

Example:
Lichen planopilaris

Guttate: Guttate lesions look as though someone took a dropper and dropped this lesion on the skin.

Example:
Guttate psoriasis

Koebner phenomenon: The Koebner phenomenon, also called the isomorphic response, refers to the appearance of similar lesions along a line of injury.

Examples:
Scaly—psoriasis
Non-scaly—molluscum contagiosum

Linear lesions: Linear lesions occur in a line or band-like configuration (Flow chart 2.12)

Example:
Linear epidermal nevus

Multiform: Patients with multiform lesions have lesions of a variety of morphology.

Example:
Erythema multiforme

Reticular: Reticular refers to net-like distribution.

Example:
Cutis marmorata fades as the skin is warmed
Livedo reticularis becomes more florid as the skin is warmed

Serpiginous: Serpiginous lesions wander as though following the track of a snake.

Example:
Cutaneous larva migrans

Universalis: Universalis refers to a widespread disorder that affects the entire skin.

Example:
Alopecia universalis

Scarlatiniform: Scarlatiniform rashes have the pattern of scarlet fever with innumerable small red papules that are widely and diffusely distributed Kawasaki disease (Flow chart 2.13).

Morbilliform: The term "morbilliform" means that the patient has a rash that looks like measles consisting of erythematous macules usually 2–10 mm in diameter but may be confluent in places.

Example:
Drug reactions (Flow chart 2.14)

Flow chart 2.11: Identification of disease through follicular lesions

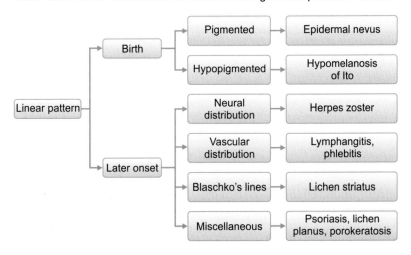

Flow chart 2.12: Identification of disease through linear pattern of lesions

Satellite lesion: Smaller similar lesion sets very close to the main lesion yet not continuous to it.

Examples:
Candidiasis
Hansen's disease

Surface changes
Scaling (see under secondary lesions)
Follicular plugging—DLE
Telangiectasia reflects thinning or atrophy of skin—Poikiloderma

Flow chart 2.13: Identification of diseases through red lesions

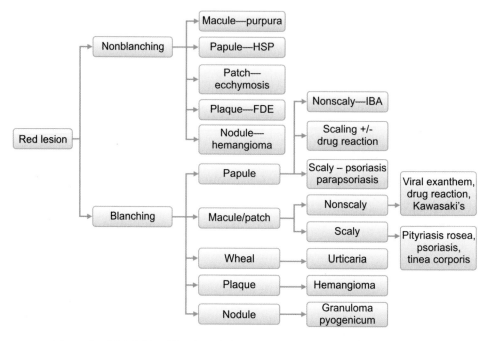

Flow chart 2.14: Identification of diseases through acute generalized rash

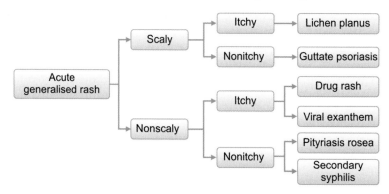

Peau de orange appearance represents dermal edema as in wheal

Punctum—MC

Dimpling—dermatofibroma

Feel

Georgetty—miliaria rubra

Velvetty—acanthosis nigricans

Nutmeg grater—phrynoderma

Sclerotic—Morphea

Infiltrated—HD

India rubber—Subcutaneous phycomycosis

Signs and special features

Some examples include:

Auspitz sign—psoriasis

Koebner's phenomenon—warts

Fountain sign—hypertrophic lichen planus

Nikolsky and Asboe Hansen sign—pemphigus vulgaris

Coudability sign—alopecia areata

Coup de ongle sign—pityriasis versicolor

Button hole sign—neurofibroma

Plummer's sign—mycetoma foot

Darier sign—urticaria pigmentosa

Pseudo Darier sign—becker's melanosis

Palpation

Tenderness

Of the normal appearing skin as in TEN

Of a nodule as in erythema nodosum (Flow chart 2.15).

Stroking leads to dermographism in urticaria (25% of normal individuals also) and urtication in urticaria pigmentosa.

Shearing pressure skin peals in pemphigus vulgaris.

Diascopy – applying pressure using a glass slide will help diagnosing conditions like lupus vulgaris.

Auscultation

For bruit in case of AV anastamosis

Examination of Scalp, Palms and Soles, Nails, Mucosae, Peripheral Nerves

Examination of the scalp

Examination of the scalp includes examination of the scalp and hair.

While examining the scalp one should look for presence of:

Scaling—Seborrheic dermatitis

Papules—Wart

Nodules—Tumors of the hair/apocrine structures

Plaques—Scaly-Psoriasis: Nonscaly – Morphea

Cysts—Epidermal cyst

While examining the hair one should examine the following details:

Pattern of hair loss and presence or absence of scarring (Flow charts 2.16 and 2.17).

Easy pluckability, as in active alopecia areata.

Easily breaking hairs (brittle hairs), as in tricho thiodystrophy.

Color of hair, e.g. a white forelock as in piebaldism.

Length of hair, e.g. differing lengths in a patch, as in trichotillomania.

Shaft abnormalities, e.g. bamboo hair as in Netherton's syndrome.

Examination should include a search for pediculi, nits, casts, and matting.

Examination of the palms and soles

Color:

Pigmented—Addison's diseases

Erythema—tender in drug-induced EMF, non-tender in associated liver diseases

Yellow—carotenemia

Freckling—neurofibroma

Flow chart 2.15: Identification of diseases through purple/blue skin lesions

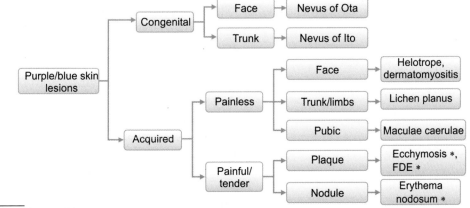

_____

*Starts red and then turns blue

Flow chart 2.16: Identification of diseases through focal pattern of hair losses

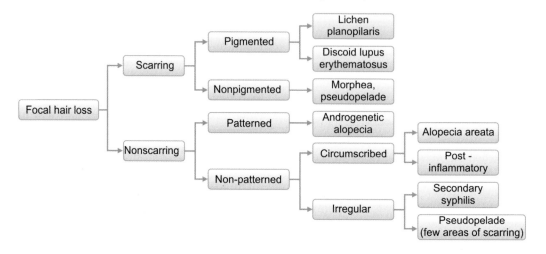

Flow chart 2.17: Identification of diseases through diffuse pattern of hair loss

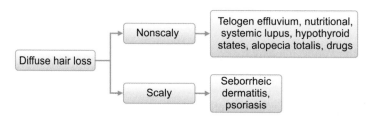

Thickening—palmoplantar keratoderma
Scaling—tinea manuum
Fissuring—psoriasis
Papule—wart
Vesicles—pompholyx
Also look for hyperhidrosis and trophic changes.

Examination of nail apparatus
Nail fold—swelling Paronychia
Plate-pitting—psoriasis
Subungual hyperkeratosis—psoriasis, Tinea unguium
Finger tip—stellate scar-scleroderma

Examination of the oral cavity/mucosae
Microstomia—PSS
Angle of mouth—perleche

Lip—scaling, as in cheilosis
Inflammation with scaling chelitis
Depigmentation and adherent scaling DLE
Gingiva—hyperplasia, as in certain drugs
Dental pit—tuberous sclerosis
White lacy pattern on cheek—LP
Tongue-White patch—Removable-candida; non-removable-leukoplakia
Palatal erosion—SLE
Other mucosae (like conjunctival, genital) should also be examined.

Examination of all peripheral nerves and superficial and deep tendon reflexes
This is important when dealing with a case of Hansen's disease or trophic ulcers.

Basic Relevant Investigations

HEMATOLOGY AND BIOCHEMISTRY

Different skin diseases show local or systemic blood changes. Therefore, blood picture may be of help to reach a diagnosis and may be indispensable in certain dermatoses. However, not every dermatological case is in need of a list of laboratory tests that may be a burden and might bother the patient leading to loss of confidence in the physician.

TZANK TEST

Cytological examination from the floor of a bulla is used to confirm diagnoses of bullous diseases. In most bullous eruption the smear will show only inflammatory cells. In pemphigus, numerous acantholytic cells with large nuclei and condensed cytoplasm are found. In herpes simplex, zoster and varicella lesions, the smear shows large, multi-nucleated giant cells.

EXAMINATION OF SKIN SCRAPINGS

This is usually used for the diagnosis of fungal lesions. Scraping is taken of the lesions of the scalp, intertriginous areas, feet, or other areas. The skin is cleaned with spirit swab and left to dry. Scrape the area with a scalpel or the edge of the slide on a clean slide. Add one drop of 10–20 percent of KOH preparation. Hyphae and spores appear as oval bodies and refractile against the background of cells and debris. Confirmation is usually by culture of the scrapping on special media such as Sabouraud's agar medium.

Similar examination is also used to demonstrate *Acarus*, lice and *Demodex*, and also for hair shaft abnormalities.

EXAMINATION OF SMEAR FROM DISCHARGE

This is done to demonstrate bacteria (gram positive cocci), parasite (Leishman bodies), and fungal grain (Mycetoma). This has to be supported by culture when necessary.

SLIT SKIN SMEAR

In all suspected cases of Hansen's disease, this is done to demonstrate *Mycobacterium leprae.*

PATCH TESTS

Patch tests are usually done to detect contact sensitizers of the delayed hypersensitivity type. Patch test is easy to apply and more safe than other skin tests. Patch testing proves only that the patient has a contact sensitivity to a specific contactant, but this does not necessarily mean that this substance in the patch test is the only that can cause the reaction but there may be other substances that may cause such reaction.

WOOD'S LIGHT

This is an ultraviolet lamp with Wood's filters, that produces a wavelength about 365 nanometers. Wood's light is an important investigative tool in diagnosis and treatment of specific skin diseases.

Wood's lamp may be used to help in the diagnosis of tinea capitis, erythrasma, pityriasis versicolor, certain pigmentary disorders, and detection of porphyrins.

SEROLOGY

This is done with consent where necessary to assess HIV status.

SKIN BIOPSY

Skin biopsy is an important procedure to confirm an accurate diagnosis for a suspected skin lesion. In circumstances, like mastocytosis and lupus erythematosus, special stains and immunofluorescence respectively may be required.

Although it is likely that the pace in the development of scientific technologies will only accelerate with time, access to such technologies may not be the rate-limiting step in cutaneous research. In fact, a strong case may be made that the limiting step will be the availability of well-characterized patient populations for study and an unfathomable clinical knowledge.

Infections and Infestations

PARASITIC INFESTATIONS

Scabies (Figs 4.1A to G)

Definition/Description

Scabies is a skin infestation by the mite, *Sarcoptes scabiei*, that is usually transmitted by skin-to-skin contact and causes generalized intractable pruritus, with frequent secondary bacterial infection.

Epidemiology/Etiology

Scabies affects all ages but is most common in young adults who often acquire it by sexual contact. In infants and young children, scabies presents with different clinical features. Epidemics of scabies occur in cycles every 15 years. Nosocomial outbreaks have also occurred. The causative agent is *Sarcoptes scabiei var hominis*. The fertilized female parasite is responsible for the infestation. It invades the stratum corneum and forms burrows where it deposits its eggs.

The eggs then hatch and continue the life cycle. The average number of adult female mites on an

---

Scabies

- ➤ Agent: *Sarcoptes scabiei var hominis*.
- ➤ Primary incubation period: 14 days.
- ➤ CF: Nocturnal pruritus , family history.
  Eruption: Characteristic burrows S-shaped, papules, papulopustules, excoriations, vesicles, urticarial lesions
  Distribution: Curve of Hebra sparing face except in infants
- ➤ Inv: Wet mount demonstrate parasite, part, product (scybala)
- ➤ DD: IBH
- ➤ Treat all contacts
  Permethrin 2.5–5%,
  Sulfur precipitate 3–5%;
  Gamma benzene hexachloride 1%
  BBE 25–33% Crotamiton 10%
  An oral antihistamine
  Antibiotics for secondary infection –
  Oral ivermectin 3 mg to 6 mg–single dose

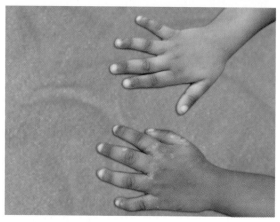

Fig. 4.1A: Classical scabies with impetigo involving the interdigital areas

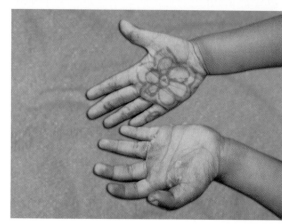

Fig. 4.1B: Pustules of scabies with impetigo

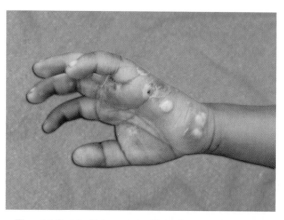

Fig. 4.1C: Medial aspect of hands are a common site for scabies

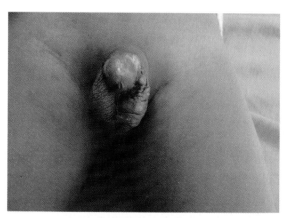

Fig. 4.1D: Itchy papules in the genitals in a child with scabies

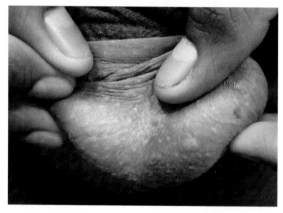

Fig. 4.1E: Persistent itchy nodule of nodular scabies

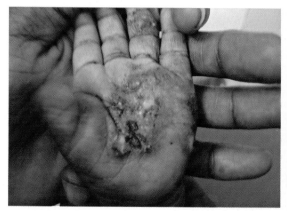

Fig. 4.1F: Eczematized scabies over the palm

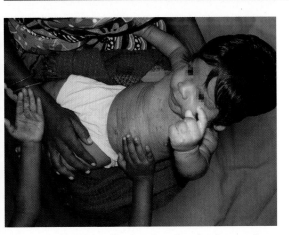

Fig. 4.1G: Scabies affecting the other family members

individual suffering from the common form of scabies is about 12. The incubation period is 14 days.

Clinical Evaluation

Nocturnal, severe pruritus is commonly present. In children contracting the infection for the first time, pruritus develops one month after infestation. In subsequent infestations itching develops within a few days (children already sensitized to the mite and its products).

The eruption is usually polymorphic consisting of small pointed papules, papulo pustules, scratching marks (excoriations), sometimes vesicles and urticarial lesions. The characteristic burrows are usually present in small numbers. The burrows are grayish brown, curved or S-shaped, slightly elevated ridges, about 5 mm in length. The point of entry of the mite, the most superficial part of the burrow, has a slightly scaly appearance, and at the distal end, there may be a tiny vesicle, adjacent to which is the female mite.

Secondary pyogenic infection may complicate neglected scabies. At times this may mask the original disease; therefore, scabies should always be suspected in cases presenting with extensive pyoderma. The lesions of scabies show a characteristic distribution: webs and sides of the fingers, anterior and ulnar sides of the wrist, anterior axillary fold, anterior abdominal wall and around umbilicus, the waist, lower parts of the buttocks, inner thighs, ankles, cubital and popliteal fossae. The face and palms are never affected in adults. In infants, however, they may be involved.

Investigations/Dermatopathology

Look with lens for typical burrows on finger webs, flexor aspects of wrists, and penis.

Look for 'dark point' at the end of the burrow—this is the mite.

Open this part of the burrow slowly and the mite will stick to the needle and can be easily transferred to the slide. If there is a nodule, biopsy may reveal portions of the body of the mite in the corneal layer.

Treatment

All individuals in the house are preferably treated simultaneously. Clothes and bed sheets should be washed or dry-cleaned. The antiscabetic preparation should be applied from neck to toes. Any of the following may be used:

Permethrin 2.5–5% dermal cream, single application washed off after 8–12 hours. A second application may be indicated a week later if symptoms do not improve.

Sulfur precipitate ointment 3–5% applied daily after a hot bath for 3–4 successive nights.

Gamma benzene hexachloride applied after a hot bath. The same clothing is retained for 48 hours and then a further bath is taken, and the clothing and bed sheets are changed. Gamma benzene hexachloride must not be prescribed to infants or pregnant women or children with history of seizures.

Benzyl benzoate emulsion 25–33% applied to the whole body except the head for three successive nights.

Crotamiton 10% has an antipruritic effect in addition to its scabicidal action. The patient should take a hot bath and dry himself/herself carefully on a towel. Crotamiton should then be applied daily for 2 days followed by a bath on the 3rd day.

An oral antihistamine may be prescribed for itching.

Children should also receive systemic antibiotics, if there is secondary bacterial infection (honey-colored crusts or tender erythema surrounding the lesions).

Oral ivermectin 3 mg to 6 mg as a single dose is found to be very effective as a scabicide and larvicide. It is best suited for treament of groups of children, as in boarding schools.

Pediculosis Capitis (Figs 4.1H to J)

Definition/Description

Pediculosis capitis is an infestation of the scalp by the head louse, which feeds on the scalp and neck and deposits its eggs on the hair.

Epidemiology/Etiology

Pediculosis capitis is more common among school children, especially girls, but all ages may be affected. Pediculosis capitis does not respect any social class.

Etiology: Pediculus humanus var. capitis. Unlike *P. humanus corporis* (the body louse), the head louse is not a vector of infectious diseases. Transmission occurs via shared hats, caps, brushes, combs, and also by direct head-to-head contact. Epidemics may occur in schools.

Clinical Evaluation

Head lice may be identified with the naked eye or using a hand lens. The majority of patients have a population of less than 10 head lice. Nits, the parasite's eggs, appear as oval grayish-white egg capsules (1 mm long) firmly cemented to the hairs. They vary in number from only a few to thousands. Head lice deposit nits on the hair shaft, as it emerges from the hair follicle. So with recent infestations, nits are seen near the scalp, but with long-standing infestations, nits may be 10 to 15

Pediculosis capitis

➤ Agent: *Pediculus humanus var. capitis* (not a vector of infectious diseases)
➤ Transmission: Direct head-to-head contact and fomites
➤ CF: Presence of lice and nits occipital, postauricular area may be masked by secondary changes
   Matting of hair - Plica polonica
➤ DD: Pyoderma, seborrheic dermatitis
➤ Treat all contacts
   Permethrin 1% rinse
   Carbaryl 0.5% (lotion – shampoo)
   Malathion 0.5% (lotion – shampoo)
   Tetramethrin 0.3% combined with piperonyl butoxide 3%
   Cotrimoxazole
   Ivermectol 3–12 mg stat

cm from scalp. As scalp hair grows 0.5 mm daily, the presence of nits 15 cm from the scalp surface indicates that the infestation is approximately 9 months old. New viable eggs have a creamy-yellow color, and empty eggshells are white.

Excoriations, crusts, and secondary impetiginized lesions are commonly seen and may extend onto neck, forehead, face and ears, and mask the presence of lice and nits. In extreme cases, the scalp becomes a confluent, purulent mass of matted hair, lice, nits, crusts, and purulent discharge, so-called plica polonica.

Papular urticaria may be seen on the neck as a reaction to louse bites.

Sites of predilection: Head lice are nearly always confined to the scalp. The occipital and postauricular regions are favorite sites. Head lice may rarely infest the beard or other hairy sites.

Treatment

One of the following preparations may be used:
Carbaryl 0.5% (lotion – shampoo) or malathion 0.5% (lotion – shampoo): The lotion is applied to the scalp for a 12-hour period followed by shampooing with shampoo containing the same

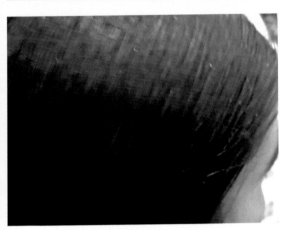

Fig. 4.1H: Pediculosis capitis showing live adult lice

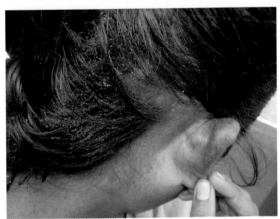

Fig. 4.1I: Pediculosis capitis with eczematisation – note the number of nits

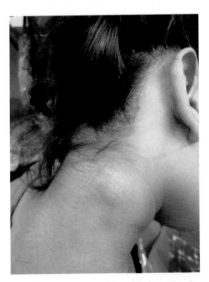

Fig. 4.1J: Pediculosis capitis with lymphadenopathy

pediculocide. Repeat after 10 days. Carbaryl and malathion preparations are degraded by heat, and a hot-air hair dryer should not be used. Unlike carbaryl, malathion has been shown to possess a residual protective effect against re-infection that lasts about 6 weeks.

Pyrethroids, e.g. tetramethrin 0.3% combined with piperonyl butoxide 3% applied for one hour and better left overnight. Repeat on the second day.

Permethrin 1% rinse (a synthetic pyrethroid) applied to scalp and washed off after 10 minutes. Permethrin is a highly efficacious agent and is much better than gamma benzene hexachloride.

Gamma benzene hexachloride is applied to the scalp and left for 12 hours, followed by shampooing. Treatment may need to be repeated. Gamma benzene hexachloride should not be used on pregnant or nursing women. Carbaryl and malathion, the acetylcholinesterase-inhibiting pediculocides, have replaced gamma benzene hexachloride following evidence of the emergence of resistance to organochlorines.

Cotrimoxazole
Ivermectol 3–12 mg stat
Remaining nits may be removed using a fine-tooth comb. Patients should be reevaluated 1 or 2 weeks after the last pediculocide application; re-treatment may be necessary, if lice are found or eggs are observed at the hair-skin junction. Affected family members and contacts should be treated. Combs and brushes should be washed.

Secondary bacterial infection should be treated with appropriate doses of systemic antibiotics, e.g. erythromycin or cloxacillin, before the application of any pediculocide.

Cutaneous Larva Migrans (Figs 4.1K and L)

Definition/Description

Cutaneous larva migrans is a cutaneous lesion produced by percutaneous penetration and migration of larvae of various nematode parasites. It is characterized by erythematous, serpiginous, papular or vesicular linear lesions corresponding to the movements of the larvae beneath the skin.

Synonym: Creeping eruption, sandworm eruption, plumber's itch, duckhunter's itch.

Cutaneous larva migrans

➤ Agents: *Ancylostoma, Uncinaria, Bunostomum, Strongyloides* - larva currens; toxocariasis–Visceral larva migrans
➤ Contact with wet sand
➤ CF: Serpiginous, migrating eruption secondary eczematisation/infection
➤ DD: Contact dermatitis
➤ Treatment:
Topical thiabendazole 10%.
Thiabendazole 50 mg/kg/d BD J 2 – 5 days
Albendazole 400 mg/d × 3 days
Liquid nitrogen spray at the progressing end

Epidemiology/Etiology

The disease may be caused by the larva of *Ancylostoma braziliense, A. caninum, A. ceylonicum, Uncinaria stenocephala* (hookworm of dogs), or *Bunostomum phlebotomum* (hookworm of cattle), *A. duodenale* and *Necator americanus. Strongyloides stercoralis* causes a distinctive form of cutaneous larva migrans (larva currens that moves much faster).

The ova of hookworms are deposited in sand and soil in warm, shady areas. They hatch into larvae that penetrate human skin. The children at risk include those indulging in sporting activities in open grounds and seawater.

Clinical Evaluation

Local pruritus begins within hours after larval penetration.

Creeping larvae produce serpiginous, thin, linear, raised, tunnel-like erythematous lesions 2 to 3 mm wide containing serous fluid. Several or many lesions may be present depending on the number of penetrating larvae. Larvae move a few millimeters to many millimeters daily, confined to an area several centimeters in diameter. The lesions occur on exposed sites, most commonly the feet and buttocks.

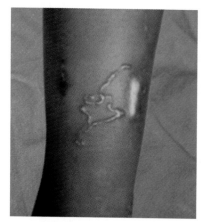

Fig. 4.1K: Serpiginous, migrating eruption of cutaneous larva migrans

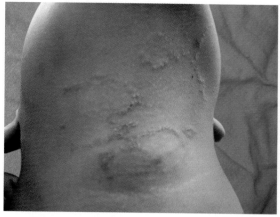

Fig. 4.1L: Multiple tracks of larva migrans

Larva currens is a variant caused by *Strongyloides stercoralis*. Papules, urticaria and papulovesicles are seen at the site of larval penetration, associated with intense pruritus. Larva currens occurs on the skin around the anus, buttocks, thighs, back, shoulders, and abdomen. The pruritus and eruption disappear when the larvae enter blood vessels and migrate to intestinal mucosa.

Visceral larva migrans (toxocariasis) is characterized by persistent hypereosinophilia, hepatomegaly, and frequently, pneumonitis. Generalized pruritus and urticarial or papular eruptions of the trunk and legs are the most frequently reported cutaneous manifestations. Rarely, a migrating panniculitis may occur. Visceral larva migrans is caused by *Toxocara canis, T. cati* and *T. leonensis*, the common roundworms of dogs, cats, and wild carnivores.

Treatment

The treatment of choice is the topical application of thiabendazole 10%. Oral thiabendazole 50 mg per kg body weight per day in 2 doses (maximum 3 g/day) for 2 to 5 days is less effective and more toxic. Albendazole 400 mg daily by mouth for three days is safe and often effective. Liquid nitrogen may be applied to the progressing end of larval burrow.

Papular Urticaria (Figs 4.1M and N)
Definition/Description

Papular urticaria is a reaction pattern to insect bites most commonly affecting children. Crops of very itchy red bumps, 0.2 – 2 cm in diameter, appear every few days. Sometimes, each spot develops a fluid-filled blister. It is sometimes called "insect bite allergy". In infants, it is given the name strophulus infantum and in the more chronic states, called lichen urticatus.

Epidemiology/Etiology

Papular urticaria is more common in winter. It may clear up on holiday or on moving house. One

> ## Papular urticaria
>
> ➤ Reaction pattern to insect bites "insect bite allergy"
> ➤ common in winter. self-limiting course
> ➤ Exposed sites – arms and legs
> ➤ Marker of atopy
> ➤ CF: Weals surmounted by vesicle
> Secondary infection, eczematization
> DD: Scabies
> *Treatment:*
> Counseling , prevention, reassurance topical antipruritics (Crotamiton), oral antihistamines, antibiotics if needed

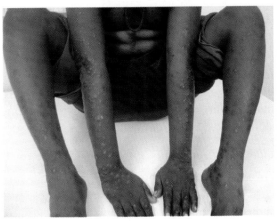

Fig. 4.1M: Child with papular urticaria – note involvement of exposed areas only

or several members of the family may be affected. Occasionally, the eruption can clear up for years and then recur unexpectedly. It is not associated with any internal complaint and is never a serious disease. Papular urticaria is thought to be an allergic reaction to insects in the environment. Often after a few years, the child becomes desensitized to these insects and the reaction dies down. A bite is not usually noticed, and it is thought that the reaction can occur simply from skin contact with parts of the insect, such as its feces and eggs — this accounts for spots in unexpected places. The most common identified causes are mosquitoes. It can

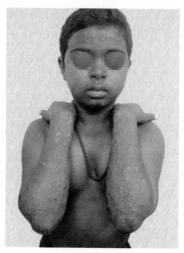

Fig. 4.1N: Cushingoid features in the child shown in Figure 4.1M and treated with systemic steroid

be nearly impossible to work out what a patient is reacting to. There have been reports of allergy to bird mites, carpet beetles, caterpillars, and insects that live in masonry disturbed by renovation. Quite often there exists an atopic background.

Clinical Evaluation

They are most often on the legs and other un-covered areas, such as forearms and face, but sometimes, they are scattered in small groups all over the body. The lesions are erythematous weals. It is difficult not to scratch the spots, which become crusted and may get infected—they are then purulent and sore. Sometimes, one new spot provokes all the old ones to come up again and itch intensely. The spots seem to remain for a few days to a few weeks and can leave persis-tent marks or scars, especially if they have been scratched deeply. Recurrence is the hallmark, and itching is very disturbing.

Treatment

This is directed essentially towards prevention. All measures possible, such as nets, covered clothing, and repellants, may prove futile. Treatment is then aimed at topical antipruritics (crotamiton), oral antihistamines, and antibiotics if needed. Coun-seling forms a major portion of management with the parents be reassured of the disorder's self-limiting course.

BACTERIAL INFECTIONS

Impetigo Contagiosa (Figs 4.2A to C)

Definition/Description

Impetigo contagiosa is a contagious acute pyo-genic infection, which is at first vesicular and later crusted. It is a superficial infection of the upper layers of the epidermis and may be caused by *Staphylococcus aureus*, by group A beta-hemolyt-ic streptococci, or by both.

Epidemiology/Etiology

Impetigo predominantly affects infants, preschool children, and young adults during hot humid sea-sons. Predisposing factors include crowded living conditions, poor hygiene, and neglected minor trauma. "Impetiginization" also occurs on lesions

---

Impetigo

- ***Impetigo contagiosa***
- Etiology: *Staphylococcus aureus*, group A beta-hemolytic streptococci, or both
  Secondary to eczema, scabies and pediculosis capitis
- CF: Scattered and discrete thin-walled vesicles erosions, golden-yellow crusts erythema heals without scarring
- ***Bullous impetigo***
- Etiology: Phage group II staphylococci,
- *CF:* Scattered thin-walled bullae without surrounding erythema
  erosions and brownish crusts, circinate lesions staphylococcal scalded-skin syndrome
- Investigation: Gram's stain, culture
- DD: CBDC
- *Treatment of primary cause*
  Sparkling cleanliness
  Soaks, topical and systemic antibiotics

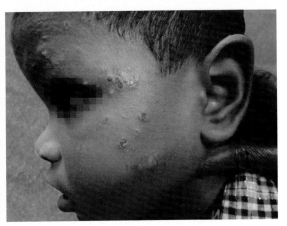

Fig. 4.2A: Impetigo contagiosa

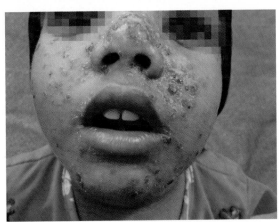

Fig. 4.2B: Scattered and discrete thin-walled vesicles, erosions, golden-yellow crusts, and erythema

of eczema, scabies and pediculosis capitis (itchy conditions). It is important to obtain cultures of household and other close contacts, and those who are positive should be treated.

Clinical Evaluation

The early lesions are thin-walled vesicles that rupture quickly leaving red wet erosions, or dry up forming gummy, golden-yellow/reddish-brown crusts. The crusts eventually separate and leave erythema that fades without scarring.

The lesions are scattered and discrete, 1 to 3 cm in diameter, round or oval, and show central healing. There may be also some large confluent lesions. Satellite lesions may result from autoinoculation. The regional lymph nodes may be enlarged and tender. The face is the commonest site, but lesions also occur on the scalp, arms, legs and buttocks.

Investigations/Dermatopathology

Gram's stain of early vesicle shows Gram-positive intracellular cocci, in chains or clusters. Use of a moistened culture swab to dissolve crusts may be necessary to isolate the pathogens. Biopsy is usually not necessary, but if done, it will show an acantholytic cleft in the stratum granulosum with leukocytes and cocci (subcorneal pustule).

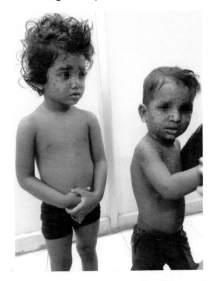

Fig. 4.2C: Impetigo contagiosa in siblings showing its contagious nature

Treatment

Systemic antibiotics: Erythromycin (30–50 mg/kg/day) in divided doses for 5–7 days or cloxacillin (25–50 mg/kg/day) in divided doses for 5–7 days.

Systemic treatment is required even when only a few localized lesions are present. This helps combating colonization of anterior nares or nearby apparently healthy skin by staphylococci. Such colonization may lead to relapses or treatment failure if topical antibiotics are used alone. The use of systemic antibiotics is also essential in cases caused by streptococci to prevent possible renal complications.

Removal of the crusts: This is done using warm olive oil or potassium permanganate 1/8000 compresses. Removal of the crusts permits delivery of a sufficient concentration of topically applied antibiotics to the site of the lesion. Solutions, such as potassium permanganate are not suitable for hairy areas like the scalp. Topically mupirocin 2% ointment/sisomicin 1% cream/fusidic acid 2% cream/gentamicin 0.1% cream or any other suitable topical antibiotic is useful. A cream is preferred to an ointment. The antibiotic should be applied 3–4 times daily.

When pediculosis or scabies is present it should be treated as soon as there is a satisfactory response to treatment of the impetigo.

Bullous Impetigo (Figs 4.2D to F)
Definition/Description

Bullous impetigo (staphylococcal impetigo, impetigo neonatorum) occurs as scattered thin-walled bullae arising in normal skin and containing clear yellow or slightly turbid fluid without surrounding erythema.

Epidemiology/Etiology

Bullous impetigo occurs mainly in the newborn and in infants and young children but may occasionally affect adults. It may occur in epidemic form in infant nurseries. Phage group II staphylococci, which produce an extracellular exotoxin is the causative agent. Phage group II staphylococci also produce, besides bullous impetigo, a rare exfoliative disease, the staphylococcal scalded-skin syndrome.

Clinical Evaluation

Vesicles that rapidly progress to large, thin-roofed, flaccid bullae with little or no surrounding erythema characterize the condition. The contents of the bullae are clear at first, and later on, they may be turbid. After rupture erosions and brownish crusts form. Central healing and peripheral extension may give rise to circinate lesions. The lesions are scattered and discrete and occur on the trunk, face, intertriginous sites and hands.

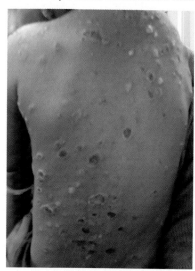

Fig. 4.2D: Scattered thick walled bullae, erosions, brownish crusts

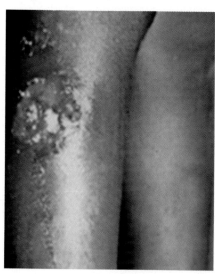

Fig. 4.2E: Deep-seated impetigo covered by crust in a case of ecthyma

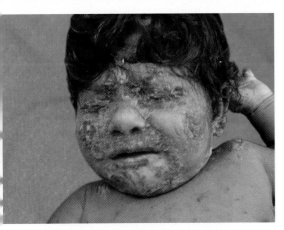

Fig. 4.2F: Impetigo over the face involving the peri orificial areas in a sick child with staphyolococcal scalded skin syndrome

Investigations/Dermatopathology

Gram's stain of early vesicle shows Gram-positive cocci, extracellular and within polymorphonuclear leukocytes.

Culture reveals *Staph. aureus.*

Treatment

Sparkling cleanliness with local and general hygiene is the hallmark of management. Mupirocin 2% ointment is effective treatment for some cases of bullous impetigo and should be applied to the lesions and to the nostrils. Fusidic acid 2% cream can also be used. Standard treatment, however, is the administration of systemic antibiotic:

Cloxacillin (25–50 mg/kg/day in 4 divided doses for 10 days), or alternatively, and if *Staph. aureus* is sensitive, erythromycin (30–50 mg/kg/day in 4 divided doses for 10 days).

Cellulitis (Figs 4.2G and H)
Definition/Description

Cellulitis is an acute, spreading infection of dermal and subcutaneous tissues, characterized by red, hot, tender area of skin, often at the site of bacterial entry, caused most frequently by group A beta-hemolytic streptococci or *Staphylococcus aureus.*

Epidemiology

Cellulitis affects children less than 3 years old, and also older individuals. The most common organisms are group A beta-hemolytic *Streptococcus pyogenes* and *Staphylococcus aureus.* In children, the common organisms include *Haemophilus influenzae*, group A streptococci, and *Staphylococcus aureus.*

Risk factors include diabetes mellitus, hematologic malignancies, IV drug use, chronic lymphedema, immunocompromise, and pre-existing dermatosis (e.g., tinea pedis).

Clinical Evaluation

The incubation period is few days. A prodrome occurs less often than commonly thought. Patients may have malaise and anorexia, fever and chills can develop rapidly, before cellulitis is apparent clinically. Higher fever (38.5°C) and chills are usually associated with streptococci; lower fever (37.5°C) is usually associated with staphylococci. Ask for history of previous treatment of prior

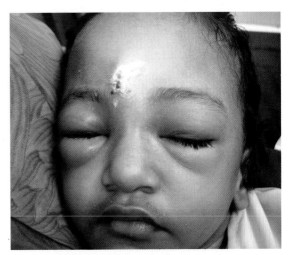

Fig. 4.2G: Diffuse warm erythematous swelling of cellulitis of the face

episode(s) of cellulitis in an area of lymphedema. The patient may be an IV drug user, and the organism may have entered through drug injection. Immunocompromised patients are susceptible to infection with bacteria of low pathogenicity.

Skin findings
Entry sites: Breaks in skin, ulcers, and chronic dermatosis.

The typical lesion is a plaque: Red, hot, edematous and very tender area of skin of varying sizes; borders are usually poorly defined, irregular, and slightly elevated; bluish-purple color is seen with *Haemophilus influenzae*. Vesicles, bullae, erosions, abscesses, hemorrhage, and necrosis may form in the plaque. Lymphangitis may occur. Cellulitis may also occur on the trunk at operative wound sites. In children, the cheek, periorbital area, head, and neck are the most common sites, and *Haemophilus influenzae* is usually the causative organism. On the extremities, cellulitis is usually caused by *Staphylococcus aureus* and group A streptococci.

The regional lymph nodes can be enlarged and tender.

Investigations/Dermatopathology

Laboratory examination of blood: White blood cell count and ESR may be elevated.

Cultures: Material for culture is obtained from primary lesion, aspirate or biopsy of leading edge of inflammation, blood. Cultures are positive in only one-quarter of cases. Fungal and mycobacterial cultures are indicated in atypical cases.

Treatment

Supportive measures include rest, immobilization, elevation, moist heat, and analgesics.

Given that most cases are caused by group A beta-hemolytic streptococci and/or *Staphylococcus aureus*, initial therapy is best directed at both organisms.

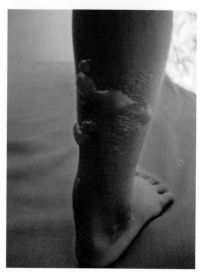

Fig. 4.2H: Erysepelas showing erythema and blisters in the advancing margin

For mild early cellulitis, if staphylococci are suspected, or if agent is not known, use oral cloxacillin 0.5 to 1 g every 6 hours. The alternative in penicillin-allergic patients is oral erythromycin 0.5 g every 6 hours.

For more severe infections, use penicillin 10 million units + cloxacillin 2 g tid IV. Ampicillin 1.0 to 1.5 g IV every 4 hours may be also used. The alternative in penicillin-allergic patients is vancomycin 1.0 to 1.5 g per day IV. Subsequent antibiotic therapy is modified according to response and cultured bacteria

Erysipelas (Fig. 4.2H)
Definition/Description

A superficial cellulitis with marked lymphatic vessel involvement caused by group A (or rarely group C or G) β-hemolytic streptococci. An interdigital fungal infection of the foot may provide a nidus for infection. The legs are the most frequent anatomic location.

Cellulitis and erysipelas

	Cellulites	Erysipelas
Etiology	Grp A β hemolytic strep, Staph aureus H. influenzae	Grp A (C G) β-hemolytic streptococci
Fever	Low/high	High
Margin	Poorly defined	Defined
Blister	In the plaque	Advancing margin
Lymphatic	Usually involved	Markedly involved
Recurrence	Less frequent	More frequent
Treatment	May need surgical intervention	Appropriate medical
Long-term penicillin	No need	In selected cases

Epidemiology/Etiology

The disease occurs equally in both sexes in all parts of the world. Release of toxins of streptococci periodically into the system induces recurrent attacks as also minor trauma or a pre-existing dermatosis, such as tinea pedis or fissured feet.

Clinical Evaluation

The lesion is well-demarcated, shiny, red, edematous, indurated, and tender; vesicles and bullae sometimes develop. The face (often bilaterally), arms, and legs are the most common sites, although not in that order. Patches of peripheral redness and regional lymphadenopathy occasionally occur. High fever, chills, and malaise are common. Erysipelas may be recurrent and may result in chronic lymphedema. The characteristic appearance suggests the diagnosis. The causative organism is difficult to culture from the lesion but may occasionally be cultured from blood. Staining bacteria by direct immunofluorescence may also identify the causative organism, but the diagnosis is usually based on clinical morphology. Erysipelas of the face must be differentiated from herpes zoster, angioneurotic edema, and contact dermatitis.

Treatment

Mild or limited episodes of erysipelas usually respond to oral penicillin, cephalosporins, or erythromycin (250 mg 6th hourly). More extensive and severe cases require hospitalization and intravenous antibiotics. Bed rest, limb elevation, cold packs, and analgesics add to the child's comfort and speed resolution of the illness. Long-term administration of oral penicillin may be warranted to prevent recurrences in selected cases.

Furuncles and Carbuncles (Figs 4.2I and J)

Definition/Description

A furuncle, also called acute deep folliculitis and boil, is an acute, deep-seated, red, hot, very tender, inflammatory nodule that evolves from a staphylococcal folliculitis. A carbuncle is a conglomerate of multiple coalescing furuncles.

Epidemiology/Etiology

Furuncles occur in children, adolescents, and young adults. They are more common in boys. Carbuncles occur predominantly in men, and usually in middle or old age.

Predisposing factors include chronic staphylococcal carrier state in nares or perineum, friction of collars or belts, obesity, excessive sweating, bactericidal defects (e.g. in chronic granulomatosis, defects in chemotaxis, hyper-IgE syndrome), malnutrition and diabetes mellitus. Furuncles and carbuncles may also complicate scabies, pediculosis, or abrasions.

Clinical Evaluation

A furuncle appears as a bright-red, tender, indurated, round, follicular nodule evolving into a fluctuant abscess, with central suppuration and

Furuncles and carbuncles

Furuncles	Carbuncles
Single deep follicle	Multiple coalescing furuncles
Children, adolescents	Middle, old age
Bright-red, tender, indurated, round, follicular nodule	Conglomerate of multiple coalescing furuncles, with separate "heads"
Diabetes less common	Diabetes more common

necrotic plug. The abscess may rupture discharging purulent, necrotic debris, and forming an ulcer with an erythematous halo. The ulcer then heals leaving a scar. There may be an isolated single lesion, or a few, scattered, discrete lesions. The lesions occur only where there are hair follicles and in areas subject to friction and sweating, e.g. nose, neck, face, axillae and buttocks.

A carbuncle is a conglomerate of multiple coalescing furuncles, with separate "heads." In the initial stage of the infection, a carbuncle appears as a red, tender, hard, dome-shaped nodule, rapidly increasing in size to reach a diameter of 3 to 10 cm or more. Suppuration begins after 5 to 7 days, and pus is discharged from the multiple follicular orifices. Necrosis of the intervening skin leaves a yellow slough surmounting a crateriform nodule. In some cases the necrosis develops more acutely without a preliminary follicular discharge, and the entire central core of the lesion is shed to leave a deep ulcer with a purulent floor.

Investigations/Dermatopathology

Blood culture should be done in cases with fever and/or constitutional symptoms before beginning treatment. If blood culture is positive, then IV antibiotics are necessary. Incision and drainage of abscess for Gram's stain, culture, and antibiotic sensitivity studies may be needed.

If the condition is recurrent diabetes mellitus must be ruled out.

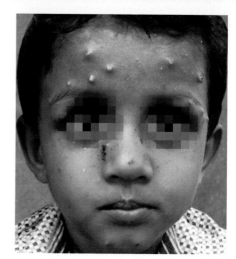

Fig. 4.2I: Multiple furunculoses

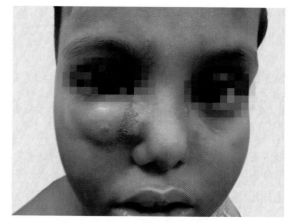

Fig. 4.2J: Furuncle evolving into an abscess

Treatment

Warm compresses and systemic antibiotics may arrest early furuncles. Cloxacillin, erythromycin, or a cephalosporin should be given orally in a dose of 1 to 2 g per day according to the severity of the condition.

When the furuncle has become localized, showing definite fluctuation, a free incision with drainage should be done without delay and the cavity should be packed with iodoform or Vaseline gauze.

In furuncles of the external auditory canal, irrigations and early incisions should not be attempted. An antibiotic ointment (mupirocin) should be applied locally, and the patient should also receive systemic antibiotics. Heat should be applied to the auricle and the side of the face. Nasal furuncles should be treated in the early stages by the application of hot saline solution compresses inside and outside the nostril, until softening occurs. They should not be incised but steamed. Antibiotics should be given internally and applied locally. On the upper lip and nose, great care must be exercised and immediate energetic treatment instituted, because of the dangers of sinus thrombosis, meningitis, and septicemia developing from boils on these parts. Incision should not be made and trauma must be prevented by the use of an adequate dressing; local and systemic treatment should be prescribed. Adequate doses of systemic antibiotics are essential.

Recurrent furunculosis may be difficult to control. This may be related to persistent staphylococci in the nares, perineum, and body folds. Effective control can sometimes be obtained with frequent showers (hot baths) with povidone-iodine soap and antibacterial ointments (mupirocin) applied daily to the inside of the nares.

Cutaneous Tuberculosis (Figs 4.2K to M)
Definition/Description

Cutaneous tuberculosis is highly variable in its clinical presentation. Depending on the virulence and number of mycobacteria causing the infection, the immunological status of the host and the route of inoculation of the mycobacteria into the skin, cutaneous tuberculosis may be classified as follows:

I. Inoculation tuberculosis (exogenous source)
1. Tuberculous chancre (primary tuberculosis of skin, primary inoculation complex, occurs in a nonimmune host).

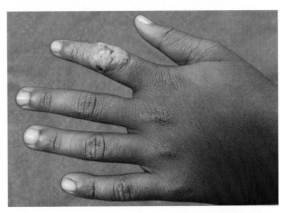
Fig. 4.2K: Hyperkeratotic warty firm plaque of tuberculosis verrucosa cutis

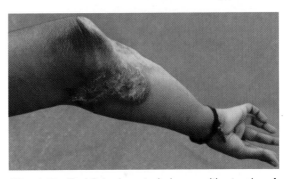
Fig. 4.2L: Reddish ulcerated plaque with atrophy of lupus vulgaris in a girl

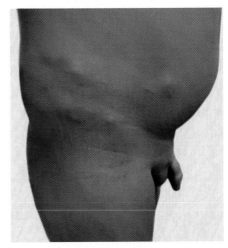
Fig. 4.2M: Erythema nodosum in a boy with pulmonary tuberculosis

2. Warty tuberculosis (tuberculosis verrucosa cutis, a form of secondary tuberculosis, i.e. occurs in an immune person).
3. Some cases of lupus vulgaris (again a form of secondary tuberculosis, i.e. occurs in an immune person).

II. Secondary tuberculosis (endogenous source)

1. Contiguous spread (e.g. direct extension from lymph node, bone or joint) may result in scrofuloderma.
2. Orificial tuberculosis (TB ulcer) from auto-inoculation.

III. Hematogenous tuberculosis

1. Acute miliary tuberculosis.
2. Some cases of lupus vulgaris.
3. Tuberculous gumma (metastatic tuberculosis abscess).

IV. Eruptive tuberculosis (the tuberculides)

1. Micropapular variety: lichen scrofulosorum.
2. Papular variety: papular or papulonecrotic tuberculides.
3. Nodular varieties (there is no universal agreement on nodular tuberculides): erythema induratum of Bazin, nodular vasculitis (some cases), erythema nodosum (some cases). Erythema induratum is sometimes considered one form of the tuberculids, but the truth of its tuberculous etiological origin is still open to debate.
   NB: cutaneous tuberculosis may follow BCG immunization.

Epidemiology/Etiology

Age: Acute miliary tuberculosis is more common in infants and in adults with advanced immuno-deficiency. Primary inoculation tuberculosis is more common in infants. Scrofuloderma is more common in adolescents and elderly. Lupus vulgaris affects all ages.

Sex: Lupus vulgaris is more common in females, while tuberculosis verrucosa cutis is more common in males.

Etiology: Cutaneous tuberculosis is caused by the obligate human pathogenic mycobacteria: *Mycobacterium tuberculosis, Mycobacterium bovis,* and occasionally Bacillus Calmette-Guerin (BCG).

Incidence: Cutaneous tuberculosis has steadily declined worldwide, paralleling the decline of pulmonary tuberculosis; lupus vulgaris and verrucous lesions are more common in the tropics; tuberculosis verrucosa cutis is a common type in Third World countries. Recently the incidence of cutaneous tuberculosis has been increasing, often associated with AIDS.

Predisposing factors for tuberculosis include poverty, crowding, and HIV infection. The type of clinical lesion developing depends on the route of cutaneous inoculation and the immunologic status of the host. Cutaneous inoculation results in a tuberculous chancre in the nonimmune host, and tuberculosis verrucosa cutis in the immune host. The modes of endogenous spread to the skin include:

1. Direct extension from an underlying tuberculous infection, e.g. lymphadenitis or tuberculosis of bones and joints (resulting in scrofuloderma).
2. Lymphatic spread to skin resulting in lupus vulgaris.
3. Hematogenous dissemination results in acute miliary tuberculosis, lupus vulgaris, or tuberculous gumma (metastatic tuberculosis abscess).

Route of cutaneous infection: may be exogenous, by autoinoculation, or endogenous.

Clinical Evaluation

Primary inoculation tuberculosis: Initially, a papule occurs at the inoculation site 2 to 4 weeks after the wound. The lesion enlarges to a painless ulcer, i.e. a tuberculous chancre (up to 5 cm), with shallow granular base and multiple tiny abscesses, or alternatively may be covered by thick crust. The ulcer margins are undermined and reddish blue in color. Older ulcers become indurated with thick crusts. Deeper inoculation results in subcutaneous abscess. Intraoral inoculation results in ulcers on gingiva or palate. Regional lymphadenopathy occurs within 3 to 8 weeks. Primary inoculation tuberculosis is most common on exposed skin at sites of minor injuries. Oral lesions occur following ingestion of bovine bacilli in nonpasteurized milk; in the past, lesions in male babies have occurred on the penis after ritual circumcision.

Tuberculosis verrucosa cutis: Initially, there is a papule with a violaceous halo. It evolves to a hyperkeratotic, warty, firm, brownish-red to purplish plaque. Clefts and fissures occur from which pus and keratinous material can be expressed. The border is often irregular. Lesions are usually single, but multiple lesions occur. There is no lymphadenopathy. Tuberculosis verrucosa cutis occurs most commonly on the dorsolateral hands and fingers. In children, the lower extremities and knees may be involved.

Lupus vulgaris: The initial flat papule is ill defined and soft. It evolves into a well-defined, irregular, reddish brown plaque. The consistency is characteristically soft; if the lesion is probed, the instrument breaks through the overlying epidermis. Surface is initially smooth or slightly scaly but may become hyperkeratotic. Hypertrophic forms result in soft tumorous nodules. Ulcerative forms present as punched-out, often serpiginous ulcers surrounded by soft, brownish infiltrate. Involvement of underlying cartilage, but not bone, results in its destruction (ears, nose). Scarring is prominent and, characteristically, new brownish infiltrates occur within the atrophic scars. Diascopy (i.e. the use of a glass slide pressed against the skin) reveals an "apple-jelly" (i.e. yellowish-brown) color of the infiltrate.

The plaque of lupus vulgaris is usually solitary but several sites may be affected. Most lesions occur on the head and neck, most often on the nose and ears or the scalp. Lesions on the trunk and extremities are rare. Disseminated lesions may be seen after severe viral infection (measles).

Scrofuloderma: The lesion consists of a firm subcutaneous nodule, which initially is freely moveable; the lesion then becomes doughy and evolves into an irregular, deep-seated plaque, which liquefies and perforates. Ulcers and irregular sinuses, usually of linear or serpiginous shape, discharge pus or caseous material. Edges are undermined, inverted, and dissecting subcutaneous pockets alternate with soft, fluctuating infiltrates and bridging scars. The lesions are reddish blue or brownish in color. Scrofuloderma most often occurs in the parotidal, submandibular, supraclavicular, or axillary regions; the lateral neck may be also involved. Scrofuloderma most often results from continuous spread from affected lymph nodes or tuberculous bones (phalanges, sternum, ribs) or joints.

Clinical features of cutaneous TB

	TBVC	LV	Scrofuloderma
Source	Exogenous	Exo & endogenous	Endogenous
Immunitry	Good	Good – poor	Poor
Site	Extremities	Head and neck	Neck, axilla, groin
CF	Hyperkeratotic, warty, firm, plaque	Reddish plaque	Firm SC nodule
Important finding	Pus from crypts — on pressure	Diascopy Apple jelly nodule	Sinus tract on probing
Lymphadenopathy	Nil	Present	Underlying

Metastatic tuberculous abscess (tuberculous gumma): There is a nontender, "cold," fluctuant subcutaneous abscess. The lesion coalesces with the overlying skin, breaks down and forms fistulas and ulcers. The color of the overlying skin is initially that of the normal skin; later, it becomes reddish blue. Single or multiple lesions may occur, often at sites of previous trauma.

Acute miliary tuberculosis: Presents as an exanthem. Lesions are disseminated and consist of minute macules and papules or purpuric lesions. Sometimes, vesicular and crusted lesions are observed. Removal of crust reveals umbilication. Lesions are red or purpuric in color. They are disseminated on all parts of the body, particularly the trunk.

Orificial tuberculosis: A small yellowish nodule on mucosa breaks down to form a painful circular or irregular ulcer with undermined borders and pseudomembranous material, yellowish tubercles and eroded vessels at its base. The ulcer is red, hemorrhagic, and purulent. The surrounding mucosa is swollen, edematous, and inflamed. Since orificial tuberculosis results from autoinoculation of mycobacteria from progressive tuberculosis of internal organs, orificial tuberculosis is usually found on the oral, pharyngeal (pulmonary tuberculosis), vulvar (genitourinary tuberculosis), and anal (intestinal tuberculosis) mucous membranes. Lesions may be single or multiple, and in the mouth most often occur on the tongue, soft and hard palates, or lips. Orificial tuberculosis may occur in a tooth socket following tooth extraction.

The tuberculids: It has been postulated that tuberculids are the result of hypersensitivity reaction to hematogenous dissemination of tubercle bacilli or their toxin in patients with moderate or high degree of immunity. Usually no identifiable focus of active tuberculosis can be detected and the tissue culture for acid-fast bacilli is often negative.

There is still much controversy about these conditions.

Lichen scrofulosorum: This is a rare form of tuberculid, presenting with grouped lichenoid papules with perifollicular pattern over the trunk. It is frequently found in children or young adults and may be associated with tuberculosis of lymph node, bone or joint. The lesions often involute slowly in months without scar and then recur. This condition must be differentiated from lichenoid drug eruption, lichen nitidus, keratosis spinulosa, sarcoidosis, lichenoid syphilis and eruptive syringoma.

Papulonecrotic tuberculid: This condition usually presents with symmetrical crops of papular eruption that proceed to central necrosis, ulceration and depressed scar. It occurs predominantly in young adult, most commonly affecting the limbs. There may be history or distant foci of tuberculous infection. The main differential diagnosis includes prurigo simplex, papular eczema, folliculitis, leukocytoclastic vasculitis, pityriasis lichenoides et varioliformis acuta and secondary syphilis.

Erythema induratum (Bazin): This is a nodular tuberculid presenting with indolent inflamed deep-seated nodule and plaque, occurring bilaterally over the calves or feet. In severe cases there may be necrosis, ulceration, depressed scar and pigmentation. It is more common in females than in males. Usually there is no evidence of other distant tuberculous foci. The main differential diagnosis is erythema nodosum (front of legs, i.e. shins) and other forms of nodular vasculitis.

Investigations/Dermatopathology

Dermatopathology

Primary inoculation tuberculosis: Initially nonspecific inflammation; after 3 to 6 weeks, epithelioid cells, Langhans' giant cells, lymphocytes, caseation necrosis.

Acute miliary tuberculosis: Nonspecific inflammation and vasculitis are observed.

All other forms of cutaneous tuberculosis show more or less typical tuberculous histopathology; tuberculosis verrucosa cutis is characterized by massive pseudo epitheliomatous hyperplasia of epidermis and abscesses.

Mycobacteria are found in primary inoculation tuberculosis, scrofuloderma, acute miliary tuberculosis, metastatic tuberculosis abscess, and orificial tuberculosis but only with difficulty or not at all in lupus vulgaris and tuberculosis verrucosa cutis.

Culture yields mycobacteria (also from lesions of lupus vulgaris and tuberculosis verrucosa cutis).

Skin testing

Primary inoculation tuberculosis: Patient converts from intradermal skin test negative to positive during the first weeks of the infection.

Acute miliary tuberculosis: Skin testing is usually negative.

Scrofuloderma and metastatic tuberculosis abscess: Skin testing may be negative or positive depending on state of immunity.

Lupus vulgaris and tuberculosis verrucosa cutis: Skin testing is positive.

Treatment

The treatment of cutaneous tuberculosis is the same as that of tuberculosis elsewhere in the body. The 2 months of four drugs and 2 months of two drugs holds good and gives successful results. The reader is, however, advised to refer to the chapter on tuberculosis for further information on treatment.

Hansen's Disease (Figs 4.2N and O)
Definition/Description

Leprosy is a chronic granulomatous disease principally affecting the peripheral nerves and the skin. Leprosy is caused by infection with *Mycobacterium leprae*.

Epidemiology/Etiology

The earliest description of leprosy comes from India around 600 BCE. Armauer Hansen discovered *M. leprae* in Norway in 1873. Humans are the primary reservoir of *M. leprae*, 9-banded armadillos, chimpanzees, and mangabey monkeys are some of the animal reservoirs. The infection is transmitted by aerosol spread from infected nasal secretions. The disease has a long incubation period from 6 months to 40 years or longer. Clinical presentation of the disease is influenced by the host immune system. Strong cell-me-

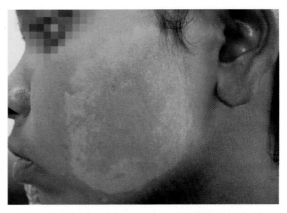

Fig. 4.2N: Hypopigmented anesthetic patch of Hansen's disease

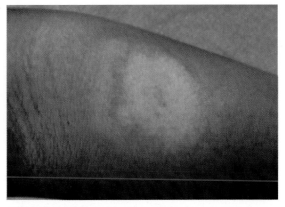

Fig. 4.2O: Type I lepra reaction – note erythema and mild scaling of the hypopigmented plaque of Hansen's disease

Hansen's disease

➢ Etiology: *M. leprae*

Incubation period: 6 months ≥ 40 years

Transmission: Aerosol from infective nasal secretion,

CF: Diagnostic criteria, out of which 2 out of the first 3 or the fourth alone is diagnostic of the disease

Hypopigmented patch

Hypo/Anesthetic patch

Thickened peripheral nerves

Demonstration of acid-fast bacilli on skin smears or biopsy material

➢ *Reactions in Leprosy*

Type I Upgrading (BT, BB, BL, LL)

• In patient on treatment

• No appearance of new lesions, patch of anesthesia, nerve thickening

• Some of the old lesions become erythematous or scaly

Type I Downgrading (TT, BT, BB, BL)

• Untreated patient

• Appearance of new lesions, patch of anesthesia, nerve thickening

• All old lesions become erythematous or scaly

Type II reaction – (BL, LL) rare in children and has a shorter course

Severe constitutional symptoms, neuritis and involvement of eyes, testes, and internal organs

Skin showing crops of evanescent, erythematous, tender, nodules, on the extremities that rarely ulcerates

diated immunity (interferon-gamma, interleukin [IL]–2) and a weak humoral response results in mild forms of disease (tuberculoid spectrum), whereas strong humoral response (IL-4, IL-10) but relatively absent cell-mediated immunity results in lepromatous spectrum. Toll-like receptors (TLRs), IL-1β (TNF)–α/IL-10 secretion, may also play a role in the pathogenesis of leprosy. A sudden alteration in T-cell immunity and activation of TNF-α with immune complex deposition result in type I and type II lepra reactions respectively.

Clinical Evaluation

Leprosy is rare in infants. Children appear to be most susceptible to leprosy and tend to have the tuberculoid form. Indeterminate forms are challenge to clinicians and have to be born in mind while examining all hypopigmented patch in a child.

The followings are the diagnostic criteria, out of which, 2 out of the first 3, or the fourth alone is diagnostic of the disease.

1. Hypopigmented patch
2. Hypo/Anesthetic patch
3. Thickened peripheral nerves
4. Demonstration of acid-fast bacilli on skin smears or biopsy material.

The easy way to classify according to Ridley Jopling would be:

Table 4.1: Spectrum of Hansen's disease

No. of Patch	Description of patch	Symmetry of patch	Nerve trunk	Glove and stocking anesthesia	Spectrum
1–3	Well–defined	Asymmetry	1	nil	TT
3–10	Well–Ill	Asymmetry	1–2	nil	BT
>10	Well–ill, inverted saucer shape geographic, midline		> 2	nil	BB
Countless	Ill-defined	Symmetry/ near sym-metry	> 2	Incomplete	BL
Diffusely infiltrated skin	Shiny coppery skin may have nodules	Symmetrical	Symmetrical	Complete	LL

To diagnose reactional states: Borderline spectrum is more prone to develop type I reaction.

Type I Upgrading (BT, BB, BL, LL)
- In a patient on treatment
- No appearance of new lesions, patch of anesthesia, nerve thickening
- Some of the old lesions become erythematous or scaly.

Type I Downgrading (TT, BT, BB, BL)
- Untreated patient
- Appearance of new lesions, patch of anesthesia, nerve thickening
- All old lesions become erythematous or scaly.

Type II reaction – (BL, LL): Rare in children and has a shorter course.

Severe constitutional symptoms, neuritis and involvement of eyes, testes, and internal organs.

Skin showing crops of evanescent, erythematous, tender, nodules, on the extremities, that rarely ulcerate.

Investigations/Dermatopathology

Demonstration of *M. leprae* as acid-fast Bacillus in the slit skin smear or doing a biopsy in doubtful cases to demonstrate the granuloma will prove the diagnosis.

Treatment

Depends on the spectrum of the disease. Since 1995, WHO has supplied MDT free of cost to leprosy patients in all endemic countries. The drugs used in WHO-MDT are a combination of rifampicin, clofazimine and dapsone for MB leprosy patients and rifampicin and dapsone for PB leprosy patients. Among these, rifampicin is the most important antileprosy drug and, therefore, is included in the treatment of both types of leprosy. Treatment of leprosy with only one antileprosy drug will always result in development of drug resistance to that drug. Treatment with dapsone or any other antileprosy drug used as monotherapy

should be considered as unethical practice. Treatment of reactional state requires hospitalization, general and supportive measures, adequate anti-inflammatory drugs, and follow up to prevent deformity.

VIRAL INFECTIONS

Varicella (Figs 4.3A and B)
Definition/Description

Varicella, commonly known as chickenpox, is caused by the varicella-zoster virus. The disease is generally regarded as a mild, self-limiting viral

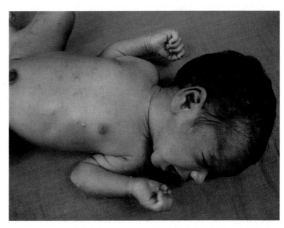

Fig. 4.3A: Vesicles on eryhtematous base of varicella virus infection in an infant. The Tzanck smear showed multinucleate~1

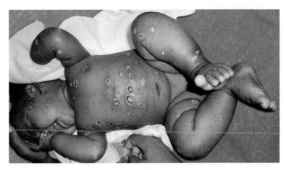

Fig. 4.3B: Varicella in HIV positive child showing ecthymatous deep lesions

illness with occasional complications. Varicella is common and highly contagious and affects nearly all susceptible children before adolescence.

Epidemiology/Etiology

The causative organism, varicella-zoster virus, is a member of the human herpes virus subfamily Alpha herpes virinae and, like all herpes viruses, is a DNA virus. The virus enters through the respiratory system (conjunctival or upper respiratory mucosa) and colonizes the upper respiratory tract. Viral replication takes place in regional lymph nodes over the next 2–4 days; 4–6 days later, a primary viremia spreads the virus to reticuloendothelial cells in the spleen, liver, and elsewhere. After a week, a secondary viremia disseminates the virus to the viscera and skin, eliciting the typical skin lesions. This viremia also spreads the virus to respiratory sites and is responsible for the contagion of varicella before the appearance of the rash. Infection of the central nervous system (CNS) or liver also occurs at this time, as may encephalitis, hepatitis, or pneumonia.

Clinical Evaluation

The following include the most common presenting symptoms of varicella:

- Low-grade fever preceding skin manifestations by 1–2 days
- Complaints of abdominal pain by some children
- Pleomorphic rash, usually starting on the head and trunk and spreading to the rest of the body
- Typically, complaints of intense pruritus
- Headache
- Malaise
- Anorexia
- Cough and coryza
- Sore throat.

The diagnosis of varicella is made upon observation of the characteristic chickenpox rash. This rash appears in crops. Skin lesions initially appear on the face and trunk, beginning as red macules

and progressing over 12–14 days to become papular, vesicular, pustular, and finally crusted. New lesions continue to erupt for 3–5 days. Lesions usually crust by 6 days (range 2–12 days), and completely heal by 16 days (range 7–34 days). Prolonged eruption of new lesions or delayed crusting and healing can occur with impaired cellular immunity.

Investigations/Dermatopathology

In general, laboratory studies are unnecessary for diagnosis, because varicella is clinically obvious. However, some tests and procedures may be helpful in confirming the diagnosis or identifying complications. Imaging studies are typically not required for varicella unless secondary complications are a concern (e.g. chest radiography for varicella pneumonia).

Treatment

Treatment approaches include supportive measures, antiviral therapy, administration of varicella zoster immune globulin (VZIG), and management of secondary bacterial infection. Early recognition of secondary bacterial infection and appropriate follow-up are major issues. Failure to recognize

---

Varicella

➤ Varicella, commonly known as chickenpox, is caused by the varicella-zoster virus
➤ Presenting symptoms of varicella are varied
➤ The diagnosis of varicella is made upon observation of the characteristic chickenpox rash, which appears in crops
➤ In general, laboratory studies are unnecessary for diagnosis, because varicella is clinically obvious
➤ Treatment approaches include supportive measures, antiviral therapy, administration of varicella-zoster immune globulin (VZIG), and management of secondary bacterial infection
➤ Early recognition of secondary bacterial infection and appropriate follow-up are major issues. Failure to recognize occult infection may result in serious illness and even fatal

occult infection may result in serious illness and even death. Isolate patients with varicella because the disease is highly contagious and airborne spread can occur. Isolation is especially important if the hospital also admits patients who are immunocompromised because their exposure to the disease can be serious and even fatal.

Herpes Zoster (Fig. 4.3C)

Definition/Description

Herpes zoster (shingles) is an acute localized infection caused by varicella-zoster virus (VZV) and characterized by unilateral pain and a vesicular or bullous eruption limited to a dermatome innervated by a corresponding sensory ganglion.

Epidemiology/Etiology

Most cases occur in individuals over 50 years of age, but less than 10% of patients are under 20 years. The sexes and races are equally affected. Immunosuppression, especially from lymphoproliferative disorders (e.g. Hodgkin's disease) and chemotherapy, and local trauma to the sensory ganglia is predisposing factors for herpes zoster. Zoster is about one-third as contagious as varicella and susceptible contacts of zoster can contract varicella. HIV-infected individuals have an eight-fold increased incidence of zoster.

Clinical Evaluation

Closely grouped red papules, rapidly becoming vesicular and then pustular, develop in a continuous or interrupted band in the area of one, occasionally two and, rarely, more contiguous dermatomes. This is what is known as zosteriform arrangement of lesions (dermatomal, along the course of a sensory nerve – zoster = a girdle, a reference to its segmental distribution). Herpes zoster lesions are strictly unilateral.

The characteristic skin lesions consist of groups (herpetiform clusters) of oval or round vesicles/bullae on an erythematous edematous base. The vesicles are clear but may be hemorrhagic. The content of the vesicles dries up after 1–2 weeks forming crusts. As vesicles start to develop central crusts, they may appear umbilicated. New lesions continue to appear for up to one week. Necrotic and gangrenous lesions sometimes occur. Herpes zoster may heal with scar formation.

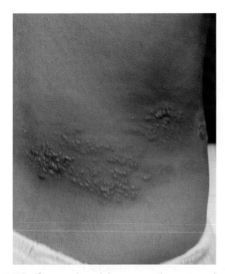

Fig. 4.3C: Grouped vesicles on erythematous base in a dermatomal pattern – herpes zoster in a 4 year old girl

Herpes zoster

> ➤ Reactivation of dormant virus (VZV)
> ➤ Common in immunosuppressed
> ➤ CF: Grouped vesicle on erythematous base in dermatomal pattern
> Multidermatomal – rule out immunosuppression
> ➤ Investigation: **Tzanck smear** to show MNGC
> ➤ DD: Irritant contact dermatitis
> ➤ **Ramsay Hunt syndrome**: Ipsilateral facial palsy, vesicles on the external ear/tympanic membrane
> ➤ **Hutchinson's sign**: Ophthalmic zoster, nasociliary branch involvement – vesicles on the side and tip of the nose

Herpes zoster treatment

➢ Disease is self-limiting
➢ Topical antiseptic
➢ Analgesics
➢ Antibiotic for secondary bacterial infection
➢ Immunocompetent: Oral acyclovir, 30 g/kg 5 times daily for 7 days, started within 48 hours of the onset of the rash
➢ Immunosuppressed: IV acyclovir or recombinant interferon α2a

Sites of predilection: Thoracic (in more than 50% of cases), trigeminal (10 to 20%), lumbosacral and cervical (10 to 20%). In HIV-infected individuals, zoster may be multidermatomal (contiguous or noncontiguous) and/or recurrent.

The regional lymph nodes draining the area are often enlarged and tender. Sensory or motor nerve changes may be detectable by neurologic examination. Vesicles and erosions may also occur on mucous membranes, in the mouth, vagina, or bladder depending on the dermatome(s) involved.

Ramsay Hunt syndrome is zoster involving facial and auditory nerves associated with ipsilateral facial palsy and herpetic vesicles on the external ear or tympanic membrane.

In ophthalmic zoster, nasociliary branch involvement occurs in about one-third of cases and is heralded by vesicles on the side and tip of the nose (Hutchinson's sign). There is usually associated conjunctivitis and occasionally keratitis, scleritis, or iritis. An ophthalmologist should always be consulted.

Treatment

The disease is self-limiting. Analgesics may be prescribed for acute pain. Topical antiseptic applications are used to prevent secondary infection. Antibiotics are only indicated, if there is secondary bacterial infection.

In immunocompetent children, oral acyclovir 30 mg/kg 5 times daily for 7 days, has been shown to hasten healing and lessen acute pain if given within 48 hours of the onset of the rash.

Immunosuppressed children should be given IV acyclovir or recombinant interferon α-2a to prevent dissemination of herpes zoster.

For postherpetic neuralgia (rare in children): Amitriptyline is useful, especially for hyperesthesia and constant burning pain. For stabbing pain, carbamazepine 100–200 mg/day is of value. Topical capsaicin 0.025%, a substance P depleter, relieves pain in most patients, but a burning sensation may follow its application.

Herpes Simplex (Fig. 4.3D)

Etiology

HSV1, HSV2: Genital (sexual).

Incubation Period

3–7 days.

Clinical Features

Grouped vesicles on erythematous base followed by erosions and healing lymphadenopathy and systemic complaints in primary infection.

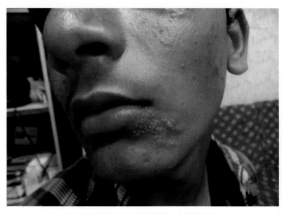

Fig. 4.3D: Grouped vesicles on erythematous base classical of herpes simplex

---

Herpes simplex

➤ Etiology: HSV1, HSV2: Genital (sexual)
➤ Incubation period : 3–7 days
➤ CF: Grouped vesicles on erythematous base, erosions, healing lymphadenopathy and systemic complaints in primary infection
HSV1: Herpes labialis, gingivostomatitis, whitlow, keratoconjunctivitis
HSV2: Herpes progenitalis, herpetic vulvovaginitis, Severe form herpes enchalitis
➤ Investigation: Tzanck smear for MNGC
➤ DD: Neonatal sepsis, aphthosis
➤ Treatment: Acyclovir oral or parenteral according to severity

---

Molluscum contagiosum

➤ Etiology - MCV1 and MCV2, Intracytoplasmic inclusion bodies
➤ Incubation period: 14 days–6 months
➤ Transmission: direct, fomite, sexual abuse
CF: Dome shaped, pearly white, discrete umbilicated papules, perilesional eczema
Koebner's phenomenon
Giant refractory MC rule out HIV
➤ Investigation: Expression & demonstration of MC bodies
➤ DD: wart, milia, cryptococcosis
➤ Treatment:
Manual removal
Topical: retinoic acid .025–.1%, KOH 10%, imiquimod1–5%, flexible collodion – 17% salicylic acid and 17% lactic acid
Electrocautery, liquid nitrogen cryotherapy, Ritonavir, cidofovir, zidovudine in children with HIV

Investigations

Tzanck smear for multi neucleate giant cell (MNGC).

Differential Diagnosis

Neonatal sepsis, Aphthosis.

Treatment

Acyclovir oral or parentaral according to severity.

Molluscum Contagiosum (Figs 4.3E to G)
Definition/Description

Molluscum contagiosum is due to infection with a poxvirus. The incubation period ranges from 14 days to 6 months.

Epidemiology/Etiology

Molluscum contagiosum occurs in both children and adults and is highly contagious. It is more common in males than in females. Infection may be acquired through direct contact or indirectly through fomites and towels. HIV-infected children may have hundreds of small or giant lesions on the face. Unusually widespread lesions have also been reported in patients with sarcoidosis and patients on immunosuppressive therapy, suggesting that cell-mediated immunity is significant in control and elimination of infection.

Clinical Evaluation

There is a variable number of small (usually 2 to 4 mm in size, but may rarely grow slowly reaching a diameter of 10 mm), discrete, waxy, and pearly-white to skin-colored, hemispherical papules with smooth surface and umbilicated center. The papules are sessile and never pedunculated. On squeezing of fully developed lesions, a white curd-like substance can be expressed. In occasional instances, a papule of molluscum contagiosum appears markedly inflamed. Ultimately, the lesions involute spontaneously. During involution, there may be mild inflammation and tenderness.

The sites of predilection include the face and eyelids, neck, forearms, trunk (particularly around the axillae), anogenital area, and thighs.

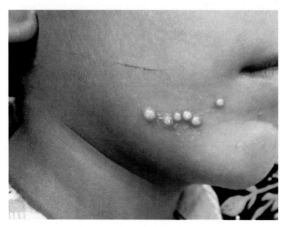

Fig. 4.3E: Molluscum contagiosum with koebnerization

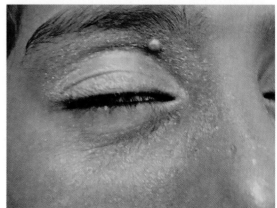

Fig. 4.3F: Molluscum contagiosum with Mayerson's eczema

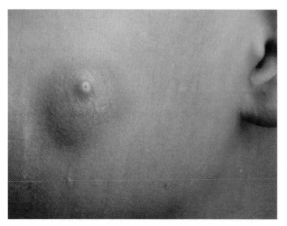

Fig. 4.3G: Molluscum contagiosum with secondary infection and inflammation

Investigations/Dermatopathology

Direct microscopic examination of Giemsa-stained central semisolid core (obtained by pointed scalpel without local anesthesia) reveals "molluscum bodies" (inclusion bodies).

Treatment

- Cryotherapy using liquid nitrogen (10 to 15 seconds)
- Simple mechanical methods like expression of the contents of the papule by squeezing it with forceps held parallel to the skin surface, superficial curettage, or shaving off the lesions with a sharpened wooden spatula, followed by application of a silver nitrate stick, phenol or strong iodine solution
- Light electrocautery.

Viral Warts (Figs 4.3H to K)
Definition/Description

These are common, contagious, epithelial tumors caused by at least 60 types of human papillomavirus (HPV).

Epidemiology/Etiology

Warts may appear at any age but are most frequent in older children and uncommon in the elderly. Warts may be single or multiple and may develop by autoinoculation. Appearance and size depend on the location and on the degree of irritation and trauma. The course may be variable. Complete regression after many months is usual, but warts may persist for years and may recur at the same or different sites. The relative importance of humoral and cell-mediated immunity is not clear. Because wart virus particles exist in the outer epithelium (granular layer and beyond),

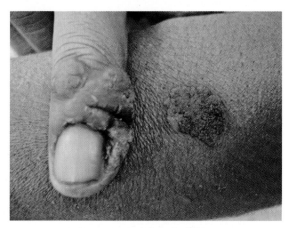

Fig. 4.3H: Periungual wart in addition to verruca vulagaris

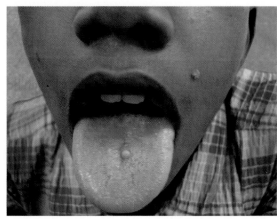

Fig. 4.3I: Wart over the dorsum of the tongue. Note wart over the face

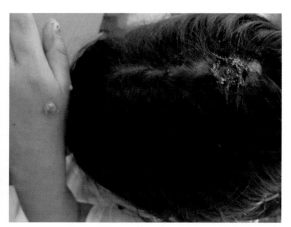

Fig. 4.3J: Wart over the scalp complicating to granu-oloma pyogenicum that is friable and bleed easily on touch

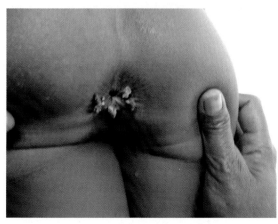

Fig. 4.3K: Perianal wart should raise suspicion of sexual abuse!

they are unlikely to become deep enough to serve as effective antigens. However, patients with immunosuppression from organ transplants or other causes may develop generalized cutaneous infections with many types of viruses, including human papillomavirus (HPV), cytomegalovirus, herpes simplex virus, and varicella-zoster virus. This suggests that some immune mechanisms are significant. In addition, spontaneous disappearance of multiple warts in immunologically normal patients who later develop lifelong immunity needs further explanation.

Clinical Evaluation

Common warts (verrucae vulgaris) are almost universal in the population. They are sharply demarcated, rough-surfaced, round or irregular, firm, and light gray, yellow, brown, or gray-black nodules 2 to 10 mm in diameter. They appear most often on sites subject to trauma (e.g. fingers,

Viral warts

- Etiology: HPV more than 100 serotypes isolated so far
- Incubation period: Weeks to months
- Transmission: Autoinoculation, direct contact, sexual transmission
- CF: Hyperkeratotic papular lesions with warty excrescences
- Common sites: Extremities, dorsae of hands and feet
- Koebner's phenomenon present
- Types:
  Non-genital: Verruca vulgaris, verruca plana, filiform, digitate, palmoplantar, periungual
  Genital: Condyloma, acuminata
- CF: Sharply demarcated, verrucous, round/ irregular, firm, papules
  Plantar wart– tender, flattened by pressure, sorounded by cornified epithelium
  Mosaic warts– formed by the coalescence of myriad smaller, closely set plantar warts
- DD: MC, Koenen's tumor (periungual)
- Treatment: Keratolytics, flexible collodion solution containing 17% salicylic acid and 17% lactic acid
  Chemical cautery: Podophyllin, TCA, cryoelectrocautery, laser,
  Topical: Imiquimod, 5FU, DNCB, bleomycin, interferon
  Systemic: Levamisole, cimetidine

elbows, knees, face) but may spread elsewhere. Periungual warts (around the nail plate) are common, as are plantar warts (on the sole of the foot, which are flattened by pressure and surrounded by cornified epithelium. They may be exquisitely tender and can be distinguished from corns and calluses by their tendency to pinpoint bleeding when the surface is pared away. Mosaic warts are plaques formed by the coalescence of myriad smaller, closely set plantar warts.

Investigations/Dermatopathology

They are not generally required as the clinical diagnosis is so obvious. Histopathology is classical with the so-called tiers of parakeratosis overlying the crests of papillomatosis, along with the vacuolization of the squamous cells.

Treatment

Treatment depends on lesion location, type, extent, and duration and the patient's age, immune status, and desire to have the lesions treated. Most common warts disappear spontaneously within 2 years or with simple nonscarring treatment (e.g. a flexible collodion solution containing 17% salicylic acid and 17% lactic acid applied daily, after gentle peeling, by the patient or parent), or the physician may freeze the wart (avoiding the surrounding skin) for 15 to 30 sec with liquid nitrogen. This procedure is often curative but may need to be repeated in 2 to 3 weeks. Electrodesiccation with curettage is satisfactory for one or a few lesions, but it may cause scarring. Laser surgery may be useful but may cause scarring. Recurrent or new warts occur in about 35% of patients within 1 year of treatment, so methods that scar should be avoided as much as possible.

Infectious Exanthem (Figs 4.3L to N)
Definition/Description

An infectious exanthem is a generalized cutaneous eruption associated with a primary systemic infection; oral mucosal lesions, i.e., an enanthem, often accompany it.

Epidemiology/Etiology

Patients are usually younger than 20 years. A large number of microbes are incriminated:
Adenoviruses
Borrelia burgdorferi
Cytomegalovirus
Enteroviruses (e.g. coxsackie viruses, echovirus)
Epstein-Barr virus
Flavivirus (dengue)
Hepatitis B virus
Human herpesvirus-6 (exanthem subitum, roseola infantum)
Human immunodeficiency virus
Meningococci
Orbivirus (Colorado tick fever)

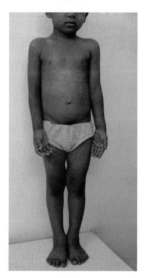

Fig. 4.3L: Viral exanthem in a child showing erythematous macular rash—anterior aspect

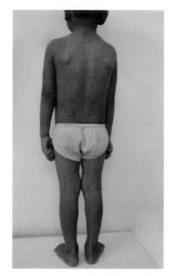

Fig. 4.3M: Viral exanthem in a child showing erythematous macular rash—posterior aspect

Infectious exanthem

➢ Exanthem: Generalized cutaneous eruption associated with a primary systemic infection;
➢ Enanthem: Exanthem accompanied by oral mucosal lesions
➢ CF: Prodrome followed by rash, e.g.
  Erythematous macules – Measles
  Maculopapules – pityriasis rosea, gianoti crosti
  Urticarial – coxsackie A9 and hepatitis B
  Vesicles – varicella, herpes, hand foot and mouth disease (HFMD), gianoti crosti
  Petechiae – dengue, meningococcemia
  bulla, pustule – SSSS
  Superficial Scalding- SSSS
  Skin Lesions are pink to red in color, usually distributed centrally, sparing palms and soles except (HFMD, secondary syphilis).
  Mucous membranes – Koplik's spots measles, vesicles in varicella and HFMD. Ulceration herpangina. Palatal petechiae are observed in mononucleosis syndrome of Epstein-Barr virus or Cytomegalovirus
  Conjunctivitis
➢ DD; Drug eruptions, Kawasaki, Kaposi's eruption
➢ Treatment
  General measures,
  Symptomatic therapy
  Specific and intensive care therapy when indicated

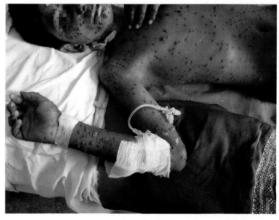

Fig. 4.3N: Kaposi's varicelliform eruption in an atopic child

Paramyxovirus (measles)
Parvovirus B19 (erythema infectiosum)
Reoviruses
Respiratory syncytial virus
Rhinovirus
Rotaviruses
Rubella virus
Staphylococcus (toxic shock syndrome)
Streptococcus (scarlet fever)

Toxoplasma
Treponema pallidum.

Transmission is via respiratory root, food, sexual contact, and blood. Enterovirus infections are most common during summer months.

Clinical Evaluation

The incubation period is usually less than 3 weeks; in case of hepatitis B virus, the incubation period is several months. A prodrome occurs in the form of fever, malaise, coryza, sore throat, nausea, vomiting, diarrhea, abdominal pain, and headache. On examination, lymphadenopathy, hepatomegaly, and/or splenomegaly may be detected.

Skin lesions: These lesions consist of erythematous macules and/or papules, and less frequently, vesicles and petechiae. Lesions are pink to red in color, and are usually distributed centrally, i.e. on the head, neck, trunk, and proximal extremities. Diffuse erythema of cheeks ("slapped cheek") is seen with erythema infectiosum. The palms and soles are usually spared, except in hand-foot-and-mouth disease (caused by Coxsackie A16) and in secondary syphilis.

Mucous membranes: (i) Findings include Koplik's spots occur in measles, (ii) ulcerative lesions are seen in herpangina (caused by coxsackie virus A), and (iii) palatal petechiae are observed in mononucleosis syndrome of Epstein-Barr virus or cytomegalovirus.

Conjunctivitis: The diagnosis is usually made on history and clinical findings. Drug eruptions should be considered in the differential diagnosis. One has to think of Kaposi's varicelliform eruption in atopic children and other immuno-compromised states with history of exposure to the varicella-zoster virus.

Treatment

Symptomatic and specific antimicrobial therapy when indicated.

The entire description of viral exanthems does not come within the scope of this chapter and will be dealt with elsewhere.

Hand, Foot, and Mouth Disease (HFMD) (Figs 4.30 to U)

HFMD is a viral illness with a distinct clinical presentation of oral and characteristic distal extremity lesions. Most commonly, the etiologic agents are coxsackieviruses, members of the Picornaviridae family.

Epidemic HFMD viral infections are usually caused by members of the *Enterovirus* genus, namely, coxsackievirus A16 or enterovirus 71. In addition, sporadic cases with coxsackievirus types A4–A7, A9, A10, B1–B3, and B5 have been reported. A brief prodrome of 12 to 36 hours duration is part of the usual presentation of HFMD, which consists of the following:

- Low-grade fever with an average temperature of 38.3°C and duration of 2–3 days
- Anorexia
- Malaise
- Abdominal pain

Hand, foot, and mouth disease

➢ HFMD is a viral illness with a distinct clinical presentation of oral and characteristic distal extremity lesions
➢ Most commonly, the etiologic agents are: coxsackieviruses, members of the Picornaviridae family. HFMD is more severe in infants and children than adults, but generally, the disease has a mild course
➢ A brief prodrome of 12–36 hours duration is part of the usual presentation of HFMD
➢ The lesions on the hands and feet are present for 5–10 days. The mucosal and cutaneous lesions heal spontaneously in 5–7 days
➢ Usually, no medical care is necessary for HFMD
➢ The topical application of anesthetics is beneficial
➢ Patient education includes good hygiene and avoidance of rupturing blisters

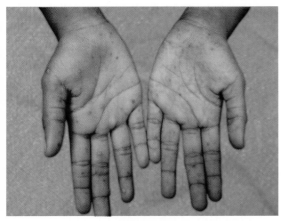

Fig. 4.3O: Vesicles over palms in hand, foot, and mouth disease

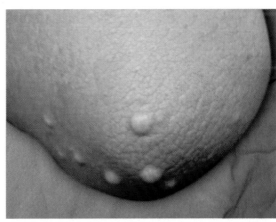

Fig. 4.3P: Vesicles over elbows in hand, foot, and mouth disease (1)

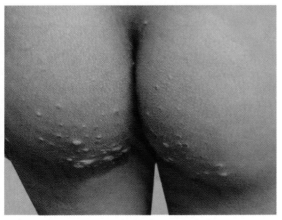

Fig. 4.3Q: Vesicles over gluteal region in hand, foot, and mouth disease

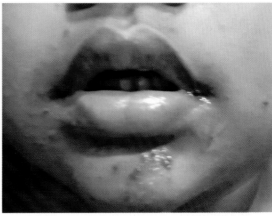

Fig. 4.3R: Classical lesions of hand, foot, and mouth disease (1)

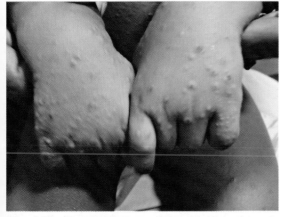

Fig. 4.3S: Classical lesions of hand, foot, and mouth disease (2)

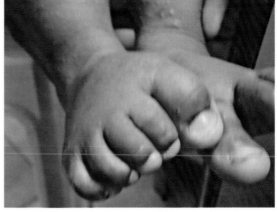

Fig. 4.3T: Classical lesions of hand, foot, and mouth disease (3)

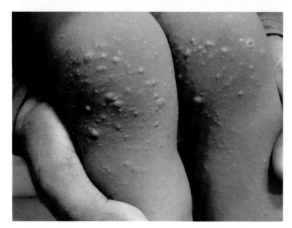

Fig. 4.3U: Classical lesions of hand, foot, and mouth disease

- Sore mouth
- Cough.

The enanthem usually precedes the exanthem that is asymptomatic, but both may occur simultaneously. The lesions on the hands and feet are present for 5–10 days, while the mucosal and cutaneous lesions heal spontaneously in 5–7 days.

HFMD is more severe in infants and children than adults, but generally, the disease has a mild course.

- Symptoms such as malaise, low-grade fever, and anorexia are often present
- Occasionally, children have high fever, marked malaise, diarrhea, and arthralgias
- Enteroviral infections may also cause myocarditis, pneumonia, meningoencephalitis, and even death
- Infection in the first trimester may lead to spontaneous abortion or intrauterine growth retardation.

Oral lesions begin as erythematous macules that evolve into 2–3 mm vesicles on an erythematous base. The vesicles are rarely observed because they rapidly become ulcerated. They are painful and may interfere with eating. The total number of ulcers averages 5–10. The vesicles may involve the palate, buccal mucosa, gingiva, and tongue.

The tongue is involved in 44% of the cases, and, in addition to the ulcers, the tongue may be edematous and tender.

Cutaneous lesions are characteristic and are present in two-thirds of patients.
- Typically, the hands, feet, and buttocks are involved
- The hands are involved more often than the feet, and the dorsal aspect of the hands and sides of the fingers are more commonly involved than the palmar surfaces
- Each lesion begins as a 2–10 mm erythematous macule on which a central, gray, oval vesicle develops
- The lesions are characteristically elliptical; their long axis parallels the skin lines
- These lesions are asymptomatic and resolve in 3–7 days as a result of fluid resorption.

A typical cutaneous lesion has an elliptical vesicle surrounded by an erythematous halo. The long axis of the lesion is oriented along the skin lines.

Generally, no laboratory studies are necessary for hand, foot, and mouth disease. Leukocyte counts are 4000–16,000/μL. Occasionally, atypical lymphocytes are present. The virus can be isolated from swabs of the vesicles or mucosal surfaces or from stool specimens and then inoculated into mice or cultured on viral tissue media. Neutralizing antibodies rapidly disappear; thus, they are usually detectable only in the acute phase. High levels of complement-fixing antibodies are present in the convalescent phase. Studies have illustrated the usefulness of a molecular assay using polymerase chain reaction primers to arrive at a rapid and specific diagnosis in order to distinguish between coxsackievirus A16 and enterovirus 71. This may hold promise in future outbreaks because infections with enterovirus 71 tend to be associated with more severe complications and fatalities. Classic histopathology findings of hand, foot, and mouth disease include an intraepidermal vesicle that contains neutrophils and eosinophilic cellular debris. The adjacent epidermis has reticular degeneration, i.e. intercellular and intracellular edema. The dermis has a mixed infiltrate. Eosinophilic intranuclear inclusions are observed with electron microscopic studies. Neuropathology in fatal cases of enterovirus 71 infection have shown features of an acute encephalitis involving the brain stem and spinal cord.

Complications include the following:

* Dehydration occasionally occurs in children with hand, foot, and mouth disease
* Rarely, complications of hand, foot, and mouth disease include meningoencephalitis, myocarditis, pulmonary edema, and death.

The prognosis for hand, foot, and mouth disease is excellent; except in large epidemics caused by human enterovirus 71 in which neurologic complications and death have been reported, especially in children.

Usually, no medical care is necessary for hand, foot, and mouth disease. The topical application of anesthetics is beneficial. Viscous lidocaine or diphenhydramine may be used to treat painful oral ulcers. Antipyretics may be used to manage fever, and analgesics may be used to treat arthralgias. Low-level laser therapy has also been shown to shorten the duration of painful oral ulcers.

FUNGAL INFECTIONS

Tinea Capitis (Figs 4.4A and B)

Definition/Description

Tinea capitis is a dermatophytosis of the scalp, the acute infection being characterized by follicular inflammation with painful, boggy nodules, which drain pus and result in scarring alopecia (kerion), and the subacute to chronic infection, by scaling patches.

Tinea capitis

➢ Etiology: *Epidermophyton, Trichophyton, Microsporum*
➢ CF: Noninflammatory asymptomatic loss of hair with broken hair
Kerion – Painful, inflammatory boggy swelling with purulent discharge
Favus – Plaque of yellowish, cup-shaped crusts with the hair projecting centrally
Easily pluckable matted hair
Regional lymphadenopathy
➢ Types:
Non-Inflammatory – gray patch, black dot, alopecia areata like
Inflammatory – kerion, favus
➢ Investigations:
Wood's lamp examination – greenish fluorescence
Microscopic examination with 20–40% KOH: for spores
➢ DD: Alopecia areata, post–inflammatory alopecia
➢ Treatment:
Clipp away infected hair where possible
Griseofulvin 10 to 12.5 mg/kg/day after fatty meals 1–3 months
Topical antifungal shampoos, creams as an adjunct

Epidemiology/Etiology

Tinea capitis affects children mainly, and adults are rarely affected. Favus (inflammatory form) may affect any age. All the three major agents, namely, *Epidermophyton*, *Trichophyton*, and *Microsporum* cause tinea capitis, although the last two are more common.

Clinical Evaluation

History: Duration of lesions is weeks to months. Symptoms include loss of hair, and pain and tenderness in inflammatory type (kerion).

Types
1. "Gray patch" scaly ringworm: Well-defined, round or oval patch covered with small grayish-white scales. The scales tend to be more densely arranged around the openings

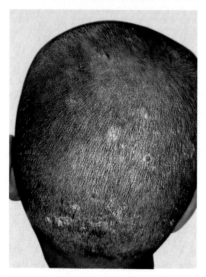

Fig. 4.4A: Noninflammatory type of tinea capitis

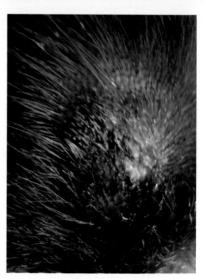

Fig. 4.4B: Painful, inflammatory boggy swelling with purulent discharge

of the hair follicles. The hairs in the affected area are broken off into small stumps. Some hairs are not involved due to the fact that the causative dermatophyte affects only anagen hair (85%) and spares telogen hair (15%). In most cases, the lesions are single or few in number, but multiple patches may be present rarely. Resolution is not followed by scar formation. Caused by *Microsporum audouinii* and *Microsporum canis.*

2. "Black dot" ringworm: Round or oval patch studded with black dots. The black dots represent the upper ends of infected hairs broken-off just at the point of their emergence from the scalp. More than one patch may be present. Caused by *Trichophyton tonsurans* and *Trichophyton violaceum.*

3. Kerion (Greek, "honeycomb"): Boggy, elevated, purulent, inflamed nodules and plaques that are painful and drain seropus. Hairs do not break off but fall out and can be pulled easily without pain (i.e. loose). Kerion heals with scarring alopecia. Caused mainly by dermatophytes of animal origin.

4. Favus: The lesion shows the so-called sulfur cups or scutula. These are dry, yellowish, saucer-shaped, adherent crusts surrounding the openings of hair follicles. A patch of favus is formed of many sulfur cups, some of which may coalesce forming larger areas of crusting with no specific appearance. The hairs in the involved area are not broken off and some of them are coarse, lusterless and erect (coconut hairs). Favus runs a slowly progressive course and may involve the whole scalp in neglected cases, with formation of scars that eventually end in permanent cicatricial alopecia.

Systemic findings: Regional lymphadenopathy may be present, especially in chronic and superinfected cases.

Investigations/Dermatopathology

Examination of scalp under Wood's lamp: Examination of scalp with filtered ultraviolet (Wood's lamp) reveals bright-green hair shafts in scalp infections caused by *Microsporum audouinii* and *Micro-sporum canis* (ectothrix). *Trichophyton schoenleinii* (favus) fluorescence is grayish-green. *Trichophyton tonsurans* (endothrix), however, does not exhibit any fluorescence.

Direct microscopic examination with 10% KOH: Spores can be seen invading the hair shaft (*Trichophyton tonsurans* and *Trichophyton violaceum*).

Treatment

Where possible, infected hair should be clipped away to reduce the infectivity of the child.

Oral griseofulvin (ultramicrosize)

Dose: 10 to 12.5 mg/kg body weight/day (maximum: 750 to 1000 mg/day). Griseofulvin should be taken after meals for better absorption.
1. "Gray patch" scaly ringworm: 125 mg bid for 1 or 2 months.
2. "Black dot" ringworm: Longer treatment and higher doses are required and should be continued 2 weeks after Wood's lamp, KOH examination, and cultures are negative.
3. Kerion: 250 mg bid for 1 or 2 months; antibiotics may be needed, if there is accompanying bacterial infection. Careful removal of crusts using wet compresses should not be neglected. Kerion should never be incised!
4. Favus: Griseofulvin should be given for 10 weeks.

Itraconazole may be used instead of griseof-ulvin for treating certain infections, e.g. those due to *Trichophyton tonsurans*, although it appears to be less effective in infections caused by *Micro-sporum canis*.

Topical antifungal preparations may be used as an adjunct to oral therapy, e.g. clotrimazole cream, econazole cream, miconazole cream, etc. Ketoconazole shampoo can be used to prevent spread in the early phases of therapy.

Tinea Corporis (Figs 4.4C to G)
Definition/Description

Tinea corporis is a superficial dermatophyte infection characterized by either inflammatory or noninflammatory lesions on the glabrous skin (i.e. skin regions except the scalp, groin, palms, and soles).

Epidemiology/Etiology

Three genera cause dermatophytoses: *Tricho-phyton, Microsporum,* and *Epidermophyton.* Dermatophytes may infect humans (anthropo-philic), infect nonhuman mammals (zoophilic), or reside primarily in the soil (geophilic). It is more common in adolescents and young adults. Tinea corporis is a common infection more often seen in typically hot, humid climates. *T. rubrum* is the most common infectious agent.

Clinical Evaluation

Skin lesions typically begin as an erythema-tous, scaly plaque, that may rapidly worsen and enlarge. Following central resolution, the lesion may become annular in shape. As a result of the

---

Tinea corporis

➤ Etiology: *Trichophyton, Microsporum,* and *Epidermophyton*
➤ Typically, erythematous, scaly plaque, which may rapidly worsen and enlarge
➤ Following central resolution, the lesion may become annular in shape
➤ As a result of the inflammation, scale, crust, papules, vesicles, and even bullae can develop, especially in the advancing border
 Sites of predilection: Upper trunk, upper arms, neck, abdomen, axillae, groins, thighs, and genitalia
 The face is also affected
➤ Investigation: KOH, fungal culture, rarely skin biopsy
➤ Topical therapy with clotrimazole or miconazole
➤ Systemic: Griseofulvin, fluconazole

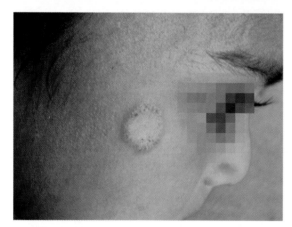

Fig. 4.4C: Annular scaly plaque with central clearance tinea faciei

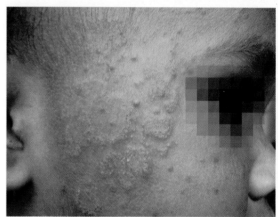

Fig. 4.4D: Tinea faciei masquerading as atopic dermatitis

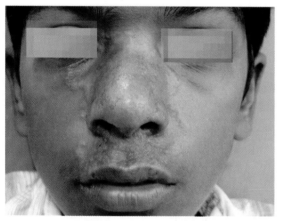

Fig. 4.4E: Well-defined annular scaly plaque of tinea faciei

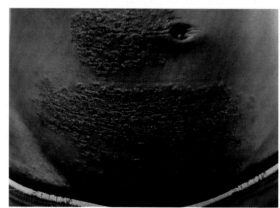

Fig. 4.4F: Lower abdomen with well-defined annular scaly plaque with extensive involvement of tinea corporis in a hosteller

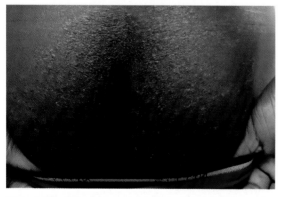

Fig. 4.4G: Gluteal area showing well-defined annular scay plaque with extensive involvement of tinea corporis

inflammation, scale, crust, papules, vesicles, and even bullae can develop, especially in the advancing border. Sites of predilection are upper trunk, upper arms, neck, abdomen, axillae, groins, thighs, and genitalia. The face is also affected.

Investigations/Dermatopathology

A potassium hydroxide (KOH) examination of skin scrapings may be diagnostic in tinea corporis. A fungal culture is often used as an adjunct to KOH for diagnosis. Fungal culture is more specific than KOH for detecting a dermatophyte infection; therefore, if the clinical suspicion is high, yet the

KOH result is negative, a fungal culture should be obtained. A skin biopsy, rarely done, with a hematoxylin and eosin staining of tinea corporis demonstrates spongiosis, parakeratosis, and a superficial inflammatory infiltrate. Neutrophils may be seen in the stratum corneum, that are a significant diagnostic clue.

Treatment

Topical therapy with clotrimazole or miconazole is recommended for a localized infection because dermatophytes rarely invade living tissues. Topical therapy should be applied to the lesion and at least 2 cm beyond this area once or twice a day for at least 2 weeks, depending on which agent is used. Systemic therapy, with griseofulvin daily or fluconazole weekly, may be indicated for tinea corporis that includes extensive skin infection, immunosuppression, resistance to topical antifungal therapy, and comorbidities of tinea capitis or tinea unguium. Use of oral agents requires attention to potential drug interactions and monitoring for adverse effects.

Pityriasis Versicolor (Fig. 4.4H)
Definition/Description

Pityriasis versicolor is a chronic, asymptomatic, superficial fungus infection of the trunk, characterized by white or brown scaly macules.

Synonym: Tinea versicolor.

Epidemiology/Etiology

Pityriasis versicolor is caused by *Malassezia furfur,* the pathogenic mycelial phase of the normal flora yeast *Pityrosporum orbiculare.* Pityriasis versicolor is considered noncontagious by many authorities. It is more common in adolescents and young adults.

Predisposing factors: Climatic factors appear to be important, as the disease is far more common in the tropics and, in the summer, in temperate climates. High levels of cortisol appear to increase

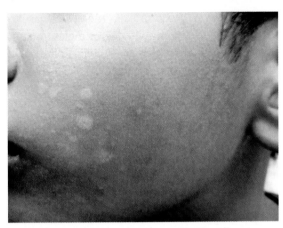

Fig. 4.4H: Sharply marginated, hypopigmented macules with fine branny scaling of Pityriasis versicolor

Pityriasis versicolor

➤ Etiology: *Malassezia furfur*
➤ CF sharply marginated, round/oval macules skin colored/hypopigmented/pigmented (pin head to more than 30 cm), with fine branny scaling positive fingernail sign
➤ Investigation: KOH or Parker Quink Ink/KOH mount – hyphae and spore – 'spaghetti & meatballs' Wood's lamp examination shows faint yellow fluorescence
➤ DD: Pityriasis rosea
➤ Treatment: Topical:
Short applications of selenium sulfide (2.5%, washed off in 30 min) × 12 nights
Sodium thiosulfate (25%) solution in water applied once or twice daily
Miconazole cream once a day
Ketoconazole (2%) either as shampoo or cream
Systemic: Ketoconazole 200 mg/D × 10 days
Monitor LFT

susceptibility—both in Cushing's syndrome and with prolonged administration of corticosteroids (topical or systemic).

Clinical Evaluation

Skin lesions consist of sharply marginated, scattered, discrete, round or oval macules, with fine branny scaling (pityriasis = bran-like). The scales can be easily scraped off with the edge of a glass microscope slide. The macules vary in color from brown of varying intensities and hues to white, hence the term versicolor. They range in size from 1 cm to very large confluent areas more than 30 cm.

Sites of predilection: Upper trunk, upper arms, neck, abdomen, axillae, groins, thighs, and genitalia. The face is rarely affected.

Investigations/Dermatopathology

Direct microscopic examination of scales prepared with KOH or Parker Quink ink/KOH technique reveals spherical, thick-walled yeasts and coarse mycelium often fragmented to short filaments. These short hyphae and round cells are commonly referred to as 'spaghetti and meatballs'.

Wood's lamp examination shows faint yellow fluorescence of scales.

Treatment

Topical agents: Short applications of selenium sulfide (2.5%, to be washed off in 30 minutes) for 12 nights. Repeat every 2 weeks.

Sodium thiosulfate (25%) solution in water applied once or twice daily.

Miconazole cream: Topical ketoconazole (2%) either as shampoo or cream.

Systemic therapy: Ketoconazole 200 mg orally daily with breakfast for 10 days. Ketoconazole can cause, on rare occasions, liver cell damage.

Relapses are very common, whatever the primary treatment, and it is better to retreat each episode rather than resort to long-term suppressive therapy. Patients should be warned that repigmentation may take several months, as otherwise they will often report treatment failure even when the organisms have been destroyed, simply because the hypopigmentation persists.

Dermatitis and Eczemas

ATOPIC DERMATITIS (Figs 5.1A to F)

Definition/Description

Atopic dermatitis is an acute, subacute, but usually chronic pruritic inflammation of the epidermis and dermis, often occurring in association with a personal or family history of hay fever, asthma, allergic rhinitis, or atopic dermatitis.

Epidemiology/Etiology

The onset of atopic dermatitis is usually in the first two months of life and by first year in 60% of patients. Atopic dermatitis is slightly more common in boys than girls. Over two-thirds have personal or family history of allergic rhinitis, hay fever, or asthma. An allergic work-up is rarely helpful in uncovering an allergen. Atopic dermatitis is also considered by many to be related, at least in part, to emotional stress.

Clinical Evaluation

Skin lesions include erythema, papules, scaling, excoriations, and crusting. Xerosis or dry skin is the hallmark of atopic dermatitis. Lichenification occurs with time. Lesions are usually confluent and ill defined.

Atopic dermatitis passes in three different phases:

1. Infantile eczema (age—2 months to 2 years): Affects the cheeks and may extend to the forehead. The lesion is an erythematous, edematous patch covered with vesicles. Eventually, it becomes exudative and crusted. Itching may interfere with sleep. There is no lichenification.

2. Childhood phase (Besnier's prurigo age—5 to 12 years). The flexural surfaces of the limbs and neck are affected. The lesions consist of itchy papules and lichenified plaques.

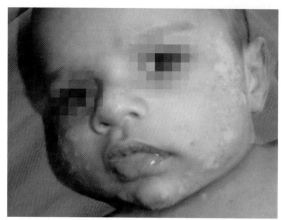

Fig. 5.1A: Dry scaly patch over the cheeks of an infant—atopic dermatitis

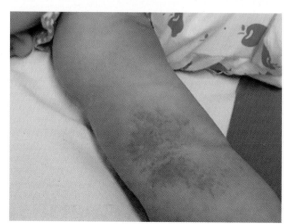

Fig. 5.1B: Erythematous dry scaly patch over the flexural aspect of elbow in an infant with atopic dermatitis

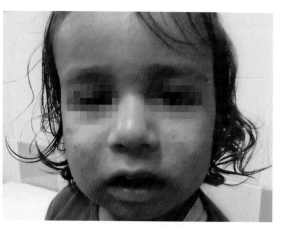

Fig. 5.1C: Erythematous dry patches in an irritable child with a history of wheeze—atopic dermatitis

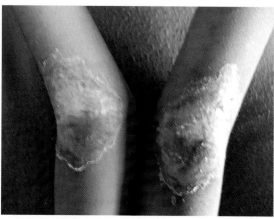

Fig. 5.1D: Erythematous scaly patch over the flexor aspect of elbows in a child with atopic dermatitis

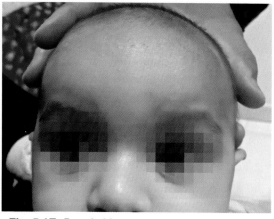

Fig. 5.1E: Dennie Morgan fold of atopic dermatitis

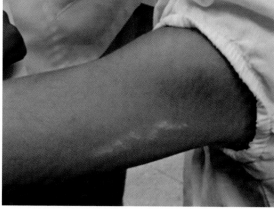

Fig. 5.1F: Lichen striatus, often a marker of atopic dermatitis

Atopic dermatitis

➤ Onset: First two months of life (by first year in 60%)
➤ CF: Dry skin — the hallmark
  Erythema, papules, scaling, excoriations, crusting, lichenification
  Phases:
  Infantile: 2 months - 2 years. Cheeks, forehead. No lichenification
  Childhood: (Besnier's prurigo — 5 to 12 years), flexural surfaces of limbs, neck — itchy papules, lichenified plaques
  Adulthood (disseminated neurodermatitis in adults)

Special features
  Tendency for generalized infections, HS staphylococcal
  White dermographism
  Bilateral cataracts.
  Ichthyosis vulgaris, keratosis pilaris
  Dennie-Morgan and Hertoghi's sign
➤ *Investigation*
  Increased IgE in serum
  Culture and sensitivity for bacterial infection
  Culture for HSV if indicated
➤ DD: Seborrheic dermatitis
➤ *Treatment*
  Education, counceling
  Hydration
  Topical: Emollients, antipruritic, anti-inflammatory agents (corticosteroids, calcineurin inhibitors)
  Systemic: Antihistamines, corticosteroids only rarely in resistant cases, for only short courses. Immunomodulators in selected cases with utmost care
  Stress management techniques

3. Adulthood phase (disseminated neurodermatitis in adults). The flexures are the most commonly involved sites; the front and sides of the neck, and the eyelids may also be affected. Pruritus is severe. The lesions consist of chronic lichenified papules becoming confluent to form poorly defined reddish-brown plaques. There is no oozing (chronic).

Special Features

1. Atopic dermatitis patients have a tendency to develop generalized infections, especially herpes simplex. Superimposed staphylococcal infection is also frequent.

2. White dermographism on stroking involved skin and/or delayed blanch to cholinergic agents.

3. Bilateral cataracts occur in up to 10% in the more severe cases; the peak incidence is between 15 and 25 years of age.

4. Ichthyosis vulgaris and keratosis pilaris are present in 10% of children.

5. Periorbital pigmentation, infraorbital fold in eyelids (Dennie-Morgan sign) and loss of lateral portions of eyebrows (Hertoghi's sign) may be present in some.

Investigations/Dermatopathology

Changes are seen in the epidermis and dermis. There are varying degrees of acanthosis with rare intraepidermal intercellular edema (spongiosis). The dermal infiltrate is comprised of lymphocytes, monocytes, and mast cells with few or no eosinophils.

Laboratory Examination

1. Increased IgE in serum.
2. Culture and sensitivity for bacterial infection.
3. Culture for HSV if indicated.

Treatment

General

1. The most important aspect of the management of a child with atopic eczema is sympathetic explanation of the nature of the condition to its parents.

2. Education of the patient to avoid rubbing and scratching is most important.

3. Topical preparations are valuable but are useless if the patient continues to scratch and rub the plaques. Topical antipruritic (menthol/camphor) lotions are helpful in controlling the pruritus.

4. Warn parents of the special problems with herpes simplex and frequency of superimposed staphylococcal infection, for which oral erythromycin or cloxacillin is indicated. Acyclovir is indicated if HSV is suspected.

Specific

1. H_1 antihistamines are probably useful in reducing itching.
2. Hydration (oiled baths) followed by application of unscented emollients (e.g. hydrated petrolatum) is a basic daily treatment needed to prevent xerosis. Soap showers are permissible in order to wash the body folds, but soap should not be used on the other parts of the skin surface.
3. Topical anti-inflammatory agents, such as corticosteroids, hydroxyquinoline preparations and tar are the mainstays of treatment. Of these, corticosteroids are the most readily accepted by the patient.
4. Systemic corticosteroids should be avoided, except in rare instances for only short courses.
5. Children should be taught to use stress management techniques.

SEBORRHEIC DERMATITIS (Figs 5.2A to F)

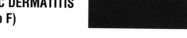

Definition/Description

This is a very common chronic dermatosis characterized by dull or yellowish-red, sharply marginated lesions covered with greasy looking scales. It occurs in skin areas with a rich supply of sebaceous glands, such as the face and scalp, and in the body folds, and presternal and interscapular regions. Dandruff (visible desquamation from the scalp surface) appears to be the precursor of seborrheic dermatitis, as it may progress through redness, irritation, and increased scaling of the scalp to frank seborrheic dermatitis.

Epidemiology/Etiology

Affected age groups include:

Infancy (confined to the first months of life) – the sebaceous glands are active at birth, but when stimulation by maternal androgen ceases they become inactive for 9–12 years.

Puberty: The majority of patients are between 18 and 40 years. Occasional cases are seen in old age.

At all ages the condition is more common in males than in females.

Clinical Evaluation

Seborrheic dermatitis causes considerable itchiness. It also gives rise to soreness and much discomfort when it is exudative and affects the major flexures. The severity and course of seborrheic eruptions are very variable, but all show a tendency to chronicity and recurrence.

There are several morphological variants, which in the adult form occur in various combinations and degrees of severity.

Infantile variants

Cradle cap (scalp).

Lesions on the trunk (including flexures and napkin area).

Leiner's disease (non-familial and familial C5 dysfunction): erythroderma appearing during the first few weeks of life, failure to thrive, and diarrhea.

Dandruff is usually the earliest manifestation of seborrheic dermatitis. At a later stage, perifollicular redness and scaling gradually extend to form sharply marginated patches, which may remain discrete or coalesce to involve the greater part of the scalp and extend beyond the frontal hairline as the 'corona seborrheica'. In chronic cases, there may be some degree of hair loss.

Behind the ears, there may be redness and greasy scaling, and a crusted fissure often develops in the fold. Adherent masses of sticky

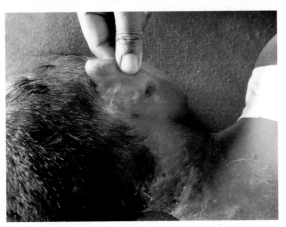

Fig. 5.2A: Retroauricular erythema and scaling in a child having seborheic dermatitis

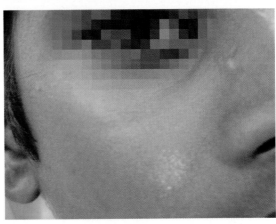

Fig. 5.2B: Perifollicular scaly macules coalescing to form patch in a boy with seborrheic dermatitis

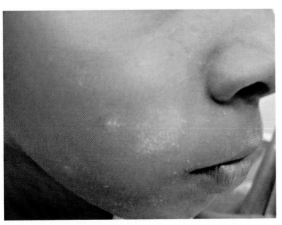

Fig. 5.2C: Perifollicular scaly macules coalescing to form patch in a boy with seborrheic dermatitis

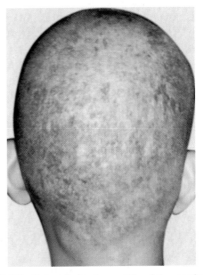

Fig. 5.2D: Seborrheic dermatitis of the scalp note the lymphadenopathy

scale and crusts may extend into the adjacent scalp. Both sides of the pinna, the periauricular region, and the sides of the neck may be involved. Otitis externa, irritable and intractable, may accompany seborrheic dermatitis on other sites, or may occur alone.

On the face, seborrheic dermatitis characteristically involves the medial side of the eyebrows, the glabella, and the nasolabial folds. Areas of erythema and scaling occur, usually associated with scalp involvement. Blepharitis is common. The margins of the lids are red and covered by small white scales. Yellow crusts may form and separate to leave small ulcers, healing to form scars, with destruction of lash follicles. Episodic variation in intensity is common, often being precipitated by tiredness, stress or sunlight exposure.

A superficial form of seborrheic dermatitis of the chin is common in young boys in the early

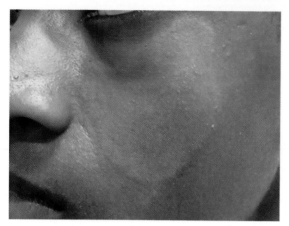

Fig. 5.2E: Hypopigmented scaly patch involving the cheek of photosensitive eczema resembling seborrheic dermatitis A

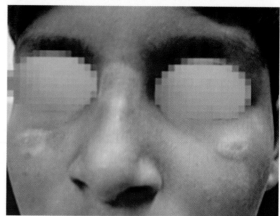

Fig. 5.2F: Classical distribution over bridge of the nose, malar area of the cheeks in Photosensitive eczema

stages of growing a beard, but it is cured when the beard is shaved off.

On the trunk, the most common form is the petaloid variety with petal-shaped lesions. It is often seen in men on the front of the chest and in the interscapular region. The initial lesion is a small red-brown follicular papule, covered by a greasy scale. Some patients have a widespread eruption of lesions, which do not progress beyond this stage. More often, extension and confluence of the follicular papules give rise to a figured eruption of multiple circinate patches, having fine branny scaling in their centers, and dark red papules with larger scales at their margin.

A rarer form, involving the trunk and limbs is the so-called pityriasiform type. This is a generalized erythematosquamous eruption involving the neck up to the hair margin. It is not particularly pruritic, and it resolves spontaneously. In some patients, the lesions may become psoriasiform.

In the flexures, notably in the axillae, the groins, and the anogenital and submammary regions, and the umbilicus, seborrheic dermatitis presents as an intertrigo with diffuse, sharply marginated erythema and greasy scaling. A crusted fissure develops in the folds, and with

sweating, secondary infection and inappropriate treatment, a weeping dermatitis may extend far beyond them. In both sexes, the genitalia may be involved, and the lesions show the usual range from minimal erythema and scaling to severe crusted dermatitis; however, chronic, thickened, dull red, scaly patches of the psoriasiform variety may develop later.

Investigations/Dermatopathology

The histopathology is not diagnostic, but generally shows features of both psoriasis and chronic dermatitis. Changes are seen mainly in the epidermis and include the following:

Focal parakeratosis, with few pyknotic neutrophils, moderate acanthosis, and spongiosis (intercellular edema). There is also nonspecific inflammation of the dermis.

The most characteristic feature is neutrophils at the tips of the dilated follicular openings, that appear as crusts/scales.

Treatment

Topical therapy
Scalp: Removal of crusts with 2 to 3% salicylic acid in olive oil is very helpful, especially in infants and children.

Seborrheic dermatitis

➤ Onset — at birth
➤ CF:
Cradle cap, eczema over flexures and napkin area
Leiner's disease (C5 dysfunction erythroderma failure to thrive, diarrhea)
Dandruff
Retroauricular erythema, scaling
Otitis externa
Over face, involving, medial side of the eyebrows, glabella, nasolabial folds
Blepharitis
Petaloid form on the trunk
Pityriasiform
Psoriasiform
Erythrodermic form
Manifestation of HIV infection
➤ DD: Atopic eczema, zinc deficiency
➤ Treatment
Topical therapy:
2 to 3% salicylic acid in olive oil, hydrocortisone lotion or betamethasone lotion/cream (avoid prolonged use)
selenium sulfide, zinc pyrithione, tar, ketoconazole-shampoos/creams.
Oral ketoconazole with caution

Shampoos containing selenium sulfide or zinc pyrithione or tar, and more recently, ketoconazole-containing shampoos.

Topical vioform—hydrocortisone lotion or betamethasone lotion following one of these medicated shampoos for more severe cases. In very severe involvement for short periods only, clobetasol propionate 0.05% scalp application is excellent.

Face: This is a difficult therapeutic problem.

Topical nonsteroidal creams, such as ketoconazole have been largely disappointing. Using the "foam" from a ketoconazole shampoo on the paranasal areas is very effective.

Hydrocortisone acetate cream, 1 or 2.5% bid with or without vioform is helpful in some. Avoid prolonged fluorinated corticosteroids because of side effects (telangiectasia, erythema, and perioral dermatitis) that can occur, even with hydrocortisone acetate.

Ketoconazole creams and 3% sulfur and 2% salicylic acid in oil-in-water emulsion-type base are alternatives to topical corticosteroids or can be used in combination for chronic resistant lesions, especially on the face and chest.

Intertriginous areas: Castellani's paint in oozing dermatitis of the body folds is very often effective, although staining is a problem.

Controlled, randomized, double blind studies have established oral ketoconazole as an effective treatment for seborrheic dermatitis. It must be noted that seborrheic dermatitis is not an approved indication for oral ketoconazole and it is rarely used in this disease for prolonged periods, largely because of the potential side effects, especially hepatotoxicity. Oral ketoconazole in high doses (400 mg) has been shown to lower serum testosterone levels.

■ NAPKIN DERMATITIS (Figs 5.3A and B)

Definition/Description

It is an inflammatory disorder characterized by the development of erythema, papules, and sometimes, vesiculation with scaling affecting usually the napkin or diaper area of infants.

Epidemiology/Etiology

Napkin dermatitis, also known as diaper rash or nappy rash, is very common. Some babies seem to get sore bottoms very easily, others very rarely, but they all grow out of it when they stop wearing nappies. Factors associated with the etiology include the following:

• Irritant contact dermatitis: Urine and feces will cause a rash on any skin left in contact for long enough. Sometimes, ammonia is formed and burns the skin.

• Infection with bacteria: Candida and yeasts.

• Other skin disorders: Psoriasis and atopic dermatitis can affect the napkin area. The nappies themselves are not responsible.

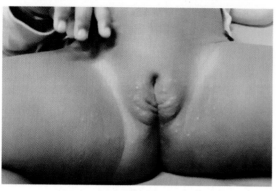

Fig. 5.3A: Erythematous papules sparing the folds in napkin dermatitis

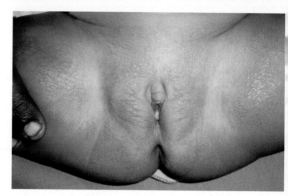

Fig. 5.3B: Erythema, vesicles, oozing, and scaling affecting the convexities   sparing depths of flexures in napkin dermatitis

Napkin dermatitis

➢ Precipitating factors:
Irritant contact dermatitis: Urine (ammonia), feces, infection with bacteria Candida, and yeasts
Other skin disorders: Psoriasis, atopic dermatitis
➢ CF: Erythema vesicles oozing scaling
Affects convexities – pubis, thighs, and buttocks
'Tide mark dermatitis' – erythematous border sparing depths of flexures
Infantile gluteal granuloma
➢ DD: Intertrigo
➢ Treatment:
Advice, counceling
Topical emollients
Antibiotics, antifungals, mild steroids

Washing powder or nappy cleanser is not either, as long as the nappies have been thoroughly rinsed to remove them.

Clinical Evaluation

The disease is characterized by the development of erythema in its early stages. This may be followed by the formation of vesicles that rupture to ooze out serous discharge. The lesions resolve with scaling. Areas affected are the convexities, such as the prominences of the pubis, thighs, and buttocks. The classical 'tide mark dermatitis' refers to the erythematous border sparing the depths of the flexures. Rarely violaceous nodules may be a presentation — the infantile gluteal granuloma — suggesting candidal reaction.

Treatment

Topical antibiotics, antifungals, and mild steroids, alone or in combination are found useful. Helpful tips to parents include the following:

• Use disposable nappies if possible
• If you use cloth nappies, use nappy liners to keep the skin dry and make sure the nappies are rinsed and dried well after washing
• Change the nappies frequently — do not leave your baby in a wet or dirty nappy
• Wash the baby's bottom at every change. Use warm water to remove all urine and bowel motions. Soap might sting, if a rash is present; use aqueous cream or bath oil instead. Pat dry carefully
• Moisturize dry skin at every nappy change. Dimethicone (silicone) barrier creams can also help
• Apply prescription creams according to directions. Strong steroid creams should not be applied to a baby's bottom.

Diseases of Hair, Sebaceous and Sweat Glands

ALOPECIA AREATA (Figs 6.1A to E)

Definition/Description

Alopecia areata is a common skin condition characterized by localized loss of hair in round or oval areas without any visible inflammation on the scalp skin or any skin symptoms. All of the hair of the body may eventually be lost (alopecia universalis).

Epidemiology/Etiology

No age is immune, but the condition is more common during the second to fourth decades of life (range 15–50 years). Alopecia areata is also frequently seen in children. Both sexes are equally affected, although some studies report a male-to-female ratio of 2:1.

Genetic, psychological, and autoimmune factors are involved in the cause, precipitation, and perpetuation of alopecia areata. The strongest direct evidence for autoimmunity comes from the consistent finding of a lymphocytic infiltrate (mainly of T-helper type), in and around hair follicles, with Langerhans cells in the peribulbar region (lowest portion of the hair follicles).

Clinical Evaluation

Typically, there is complete or nearly complete absence of hair in one or several circumscribed areas. The skin in the area(s) involved, apart from hair loss, is completely normal. There are no visible signs of inflammation, no scales, no scarring, and the follicular openings are preserved.

Alopecia areata can affect any hairy part of the skin. The scalp is the most common site, but lesions may be present at other sites, even without involvement of the scalp (the beard, moustache, eyebrows, eyelashes, and pubic hairs are not infrequently affected). The condition may progress to involve the whole scalp (alopecia totalis), or even the whole body (alopecia universalis); in such extensive cases, the loss of hair is often permanent.

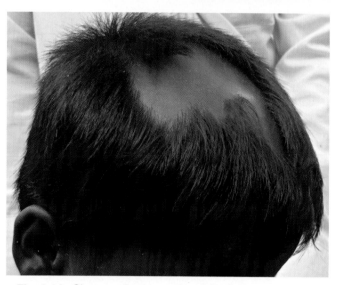

Fig. 6.1A: Circumscribed smooth patch of nonscarring hair loss classical of alopecia areata

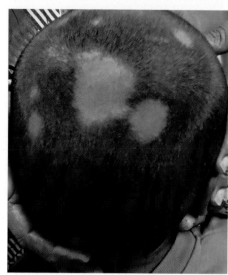

Fig. 6.1B: Multiple patches of alopecia areata

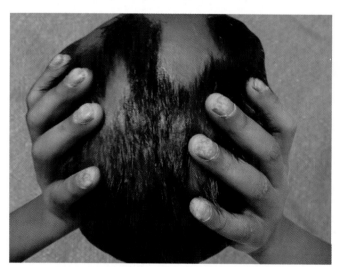

Fig. 6.1C: Alopecia areata with nail dystrophy

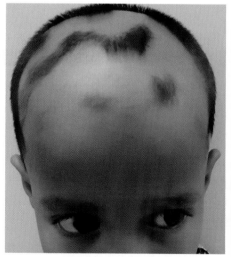

Fig. 6.1D: Alopecia areata evolving to alopecia totalis

The extension of alopecia along the scalp margin is known as ophiasis and is also associated with poor prognosis.

The size of single patches varies from one to several centimeters in diameter. A patch of alopecia areata may remain stationary in size or may progress peripherally. The presence of exclamation-mark hairs indicates progression of the patch (active disease). Exclamation-mark hairs are broken off stubby hairs that are thin proximally and thick distally.

Dystrophic nail changes occur in 20% of cases in the form of pits (fine stippling like "hammered brass"), longitudinal ridging and thickening.

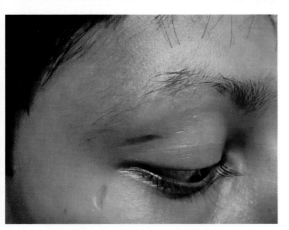

Fig. 6.1E: Alopecia areata of eyebrow and eye lashes — poor prognostic sign

There are many reports of cataracts in association with alopecia totalis.

Investigations/Dermatopathology

Hair follicles are reduced in size, arrested in anagen IV, and lie high in the dermis. A perifollicular lymphocytic infiltrate is present, with degenerative changes in the blood vessels that lead to the hair papillae. The percentage of telogen hair is increased to 25 to 40% (the normal percentage should be less than 20%).

Treatment

Local irritant applications as tincture iodine or tincture capsicum; dithranol and phenol are also sometimes used.

Topical and intralesional steroids: Topical clobetasol propionate ointment or halcinonide may be used for 6 weeks only, as skin atrophy can occur.

For small solitary patches, intralesional triamcinolone suspension (diluted 1:5) either by fine needle injection or by jet injection is also effective, but atrophy may occur.

Avoid systemic corticosteroids.

Topical immunotherapy, e.g. dinitrochlorobenzene (DNCB) or better diphencyprone

Alopecia areata

➢ Etiology: Genetic, psychological, autoimmune, infective
➢ CF: Asmptomatic, circumscribed area of smooth non-scarring patch of baldness
 Alopecia areata – circumscribed
 Alopecia totalis – whole scalp
 Alopecia universalis – whole body
 Ophiasis
 Hair pull test positive – Easy pluckability of hair
 Exclamation – mark hairs
 Nail – pits, ridges ("hammered brass"), 20 nail dystrophy
 Associated atopy – Guarded prognosis
➢ DD: Tinea capitis
➢ Investigation: KOH examination to rule out T. capitis
➢ Treatment:
 Local irritant
 Topical and intralesional steroids (beware of skin atrophy)
 Topical immunotherapy, e.g., DNCB DCP.
 Topical calcineurin inhibitors in atopy associated cases
 Topical minoxidil 2% solution
 Photochemotherapy (PUVA)
 Systemic immunomodulators, e.g. levamisole
 Avoid systemic corticosteroids
➢ Wigs are very satisfactory, especially for girls

(DCP). These are potent sensitizing chemicals aimed at inducing and maintaining a contact dermatitis at the site of application and, thus, act as immune enhancers following are also used:

• Photochemotherapy (PUVA).
• Topical minoxidil 2% solution.
• Wigs are very satisfactory, especially for women.

ACNE VULGARIS (Figs 6.2A to D)

Definition/Description

Acne is a common chronic inflammation of the pilosebaceous units that affect many adolescents during puberty. The skin eruptions primarily appear on the face, upper back and/or chest and manifest as comedowns, papules, nodules, cysts, or papulopustules, often but not always, followed by pitted or hypertrophic scars.

Epidemiology/Etiology

Acne starts at the age of 10 to 17 years in females and 14 to 19 in males, but it may appear first at 25 years. It is usually more severe in males than females, but may persist in women till the age of 35.

Multiple factors—genetic, exposure to acnegenic mineral oils and dioxin, some drugs (like lithium, hydantoin, and systemic corticosteroids), endocrine factors (androgens), emotional stress (school, social problems), pressure on skin by leaning face on hands—are known to exacerbate acne. Acne is not caused by chocolate, fatty foods, or in fact, by any kind of food apart from iodine-containing products.

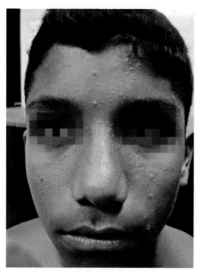

Fig. 6.2A: Seborrhea with early acne in a 10-year-old boy

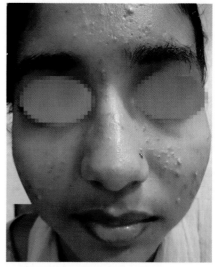

Fig. 6.2B: Comedones, papules, pustules, pitted scars, and seborrhea in a 12-year-old girl

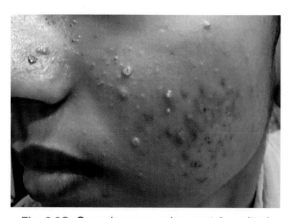

Fig. 6.2C: Comedones, papules, pustules, pitted scars, and seborrhea in a 12-year-old AV

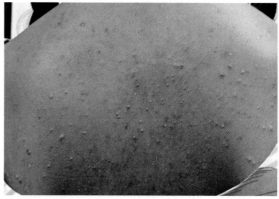

Fig. 6.4D: Comedones, papules, and pustules of acne in a prepubertal girl

Acne vulgaris

- ➤ Factors – genetic, hormonal surge (puberty), seborrhea, ductal hypercornification, *P. ovale*, inflammation
- ➤ CF: Seborrhea of the face and scalp
  Comedones, open (blackheads) or closed (whiteheads)
  Papules, with (red) or without inflammation.
  Nodules, noduloulcerative lesions, or cysts 2 to 5 cm in diameter
  Scars—Atrophic, pitted, keloids
  Sites of predilection—Face, neck, upper arms and trunk
- ➤ DD: Acneiform eruption caused by drugs like corticosteroid
- ➤ Treatment
  Mild acne:
  Topical antibiotics (clindamycin, erythromycin)
  Benzoyl peroxide gels (2%, 5%)
  Topical retinoids - tretinoin 0.01% gel and increased to 0.025%, adapelene, applied nightly
  Topical antibiotics are applied during the day
  Severe forms: Add
  Oral antibiotics like azithromycine pulse, tetracyclines, minocycline (in older children/adolscents) NSAID
  13-cis-retinoic acid is highly effective but used with extreme caution and consent from patient and parent

Clinical Evaluation

Skin lesions include the following:

1. Comedones, open (blackheads) or closed (whiteheads).
2. Papules, with (red) or without inflammation.
3. Nodules, noduloulcerative lesions, or cysts 2 to 5 cm in diameter.
4. Scars, atrophic depressed (often pitted) or hypertrophic (keloid) scars.

Seborrhea of the face and scalp is often present. Acne lesions are round; nodules may coalesce forming linear mounds. The lesions may be isolated and single (e.g. nodule) or scattered and discrete (e.g. papules, cysts, nodules). The sites of predilection include the face, neck, upper arms, and trunk.

Treatment

For mild acne

1. Topical antibiotics (clindamycin, erythromycin)
2. Benzoyl peroxide gels (2%, 5%)
3. Topical retinoids (vitamin A acid) are effective but require detailed instructions and gradual increases in concentration. Improvement occurs over a period of 2 to 5 months and may take even longer for non-inflamed comedones. For most patients, start with tretinoin 0.01% gel and increase after one month to 0.025%, applied nightly after washing with a mild soap. Topical antibiotics are applied during the day.

For severe forms

1. Oral tetracyclines added to the above — minocycline, 50 to 100 mg bid, for instance; could be tapered to 50 mg/day.
2. In females only, severe acne can be controlled with high doses of oral estrogens combined with progesterone. However, cerebrovascular disorders are a serious risk.
3. Oral 13-cis-retinoic acid is highly effective for cystic acne. This treatment requires experience. As retinoids are teratogenic in pregnant females, it is necessary that female patients have a pretreatment pregnancy test, and they must be on oral contraceptives at least one month prior to beginning treatment, throughout treatment, and for 2 months after discontinuation of treatment. Furthermore, a patient must have a negative serum pregnancy test within the 2 weeks prior to beginning treatment. Dosage: 0.5 to 1 mg/kg/day with meals for a 15- to 20-week course that is usually adequate. About 30% of patients require two 4-month courses with a 2-month rest period in-between. Careful monitoring of the blood is necessary during therapy, especially in patients with elevated blood triglycerides before therapy is begun.

MILIARIA RUBRA (Figs 6.3A to D)

Definition/Description

An acute inflammatory pruritic eruption may occur due to blockage of eccrine sweat gland ducts and retained sweats.

Epidemiology/Etiology

Miliaria usually occurs in warm humid weather but may occur in cool weather in an overdressed patient. The horny layer of the epidermis swells, obstructing eccrine sweat gland ducts. Sweat fails to reach the skin surface and is trapped in the epidermis or dermis, where it causes irritation (prickling) and often severe itching.

Clinical Evaluation

Appearance of the lesions depends on the depth of the obstruction. In miliaria crystallina, ductal obstruction is in the uppermost epidermis, and the typical

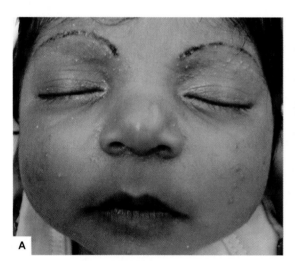
A

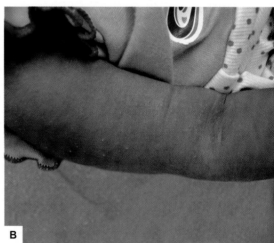
B

Figs 6.3A and B: Superficial erythematous vesicles and pustules in a febrile child—a case of miliaria rubra with pustule

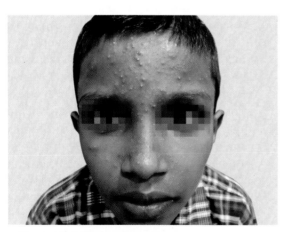

Fig. 6.3C: Miliaria rubra with secondary bacterial infection leading to periporitis

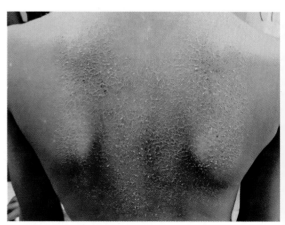

Fig. 6.3D: Miliaria rubra over the interscapular region

Miliaria rubra

- ➤ Intraepidermal obstruction of eccrine sweat ducts
- ➤ CF: Varies according to type
  Miliaria crystalline—minute tense transparent, vesicles without inflammation
  Miliaria rubra—Itchy small erythematous papule with burning sensation
  Miliaria profunda—painful larger, deeper-seated, papules facours intertriginous areas
- ➤ DD: Viral exanthem, drug reaction
- ➤ Treatment:
  Avoid conditions that induce sweating (air-conditioned environment—ideal)
  change of environment and lighter clothing
  Symptomatic (cooling and drying the involved areas)
  Calamine lotions to sooth
  Corticosteroid lotions, to reduce inflammation sometimes with 0.25% menthol
  Oral vitamin C and antibiotic, if there is infection

minute lesions are tense transparent vesicles that lack inflammation. In miliaria rubra, obstruction with inflammation occurs deeper in the epidermal acrosyringium, and the lesions are red. In miliaria profunda, ductal obstruction occurs at the entrance of the duct into the dermal papillae. It is the deepest and most severe form of miliaria. Miliaria profunda manifests with larger, deeper-seated, frequently painful papules. Intertriginous areas are favored.

Treatment

Treatment is symptomatic (cooling and drying the involved areas) and prophylactic (avoiding conditions that may induce sweating). An air-conditioned environment is ideal. Corticosteroid lotions, sometimes with 0.25% menthol added, are often used; however, topical therapy is less effective than a change of environment and lighter clothing.

Urticaria and Vascular Reactions

URTICARIA AND ANGIOEDEMA (Figs 7.1A to G)

Definition/Description

Urticaria and angioedema are composed of transient weals (at times spelt as wheals — edematous papules and plaques, usually pruritic) and of larger edematous areas that involve the dermis and subcutaneous tissue (angioedema). Urticaria and/or angioedema may be acute recurrent or chronic recurrent. There are some syndromes with angioedema in which urticarial weals are rarely present (e.g. hereditary angioedema).

Epidemiology/Etiology

Angioedema and urticaria can be classified as IgE-mediated, hypocomplementemic, or related to physical stimuli (water, cold, sunlight, and pressure), or idiosyncratic. The syndrome, angioedema-urticaria-eosinophilia syndrome, is related to action of the eosinophil major basic protein.

General types include acute urticaria (less than 6 weeks), often IgE-dependent with atopic background and chronic urticaria (more than 6 weeks), rarely IgE-dependent. The etiology is unknown in 80 to 90%; often emotional stress seems to be an exacerbating factor. Intolerance to salicylates may be present.

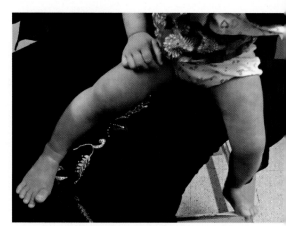

Fig. 7.1A: Acute urticaria in a child following streptococcal sore throat

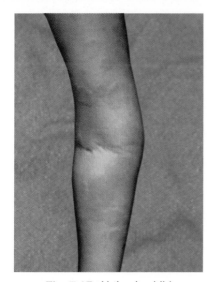

Fig. 7.1B: Urticaria child

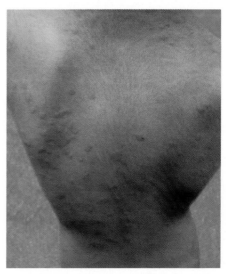

Fig. 7.1C: Itchy evanescent erythematous wheals of urticaria in case of acute urticaria due to food allergy to prawn

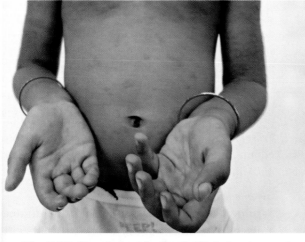

Fig. 7.1D: Drug-induced urticaria. Note involvement of palms

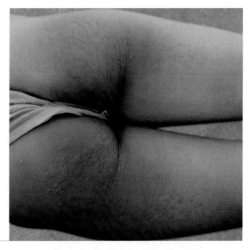

Fig. 7.1E: Pressure urticaria

Clinical Evaluation

The duration of lesions is hours. Skin symptoms include pruritus, pain on walking (in foot involvement), flushing, burning, and wheezing (in cholinergic urticaria). Constitutional symptoms may be present in the form of fever in serum sickness and in the angioedema-urticaria-eosin-ophilia syndrome. In angioedema, hoarseness, stridor, and dyspnea also occur. Patients may have arthralgia (serum sickness, necrotizing vasculitis, hepatitis).

Skin lesions: Skin lesions consist of transient pruritic papular weals — many small (a size of 1 to 2 mm is typical in cholinergic urticaria).

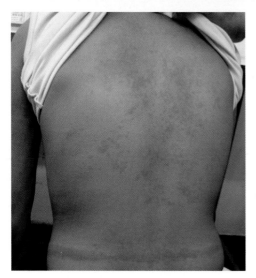

Fig. 7.1F: Combination of pressure urticaria and idiopathic urticaria

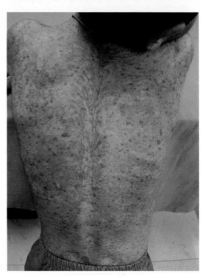

Fig. 7.1G: Urticaria in a child with mastocytosis

Urticaria and angioedema

➤ Acute urticaria: (<6 weeks), often Ig E-dependent, atopic background

➤ Chronic urticaria: (>6 weeks), rarely I-dependent; unknown etiology, often exacerbated by emotional stress

➤ Intolerance to salicylates may be present.

➤ *Points to remember:*
Flushing, burning, and wheezing in cholinergic urticaria.
Constitutional symptoms/fever- in serum sickness and angioedema-urticaria-eosinophilia syndrome
Hoarseness, stridor, and dyspnea – in angioedema
Arthralgia in serum sickness, necrotizing vasculitis, hepatitis

➤ *Emergency treatment*
Should start with injection of adrenaline subcutaneously. Hydrocortisone IV should follow but not before adrenaline.

Weals — small (1 cm) to large (8 cm), edematous plaques

Angioedema — skin-colored enlargement of portion of the face (eyelids, lips, tongue) or extremity.

Investigations/Dermatopathology

Dermatopathology: Changes are observed in the dermis, and include edema of the dermis or subcutaneous tissue, dilatation of venules, and mast cell degranulation. In necrotizing vasculitis, biopsy is diagnostic. In angioedema-urticaria-eosinophilia syndrome, major basic protein is present outside the eosinophils around blood vessels and collagen bundles. There is dermal edema, a perivascular lymphocytic infiltration, and diffuse eosinophilic in infiltration.

General laboratory tests

Serologic tests: Search for hepatitis-associated antigen. Assessment of the complement system. Assessment of specific IgE antibodies by radio allergo sorbent assay (RAST).

Hematologic tests: ESR is often elevated in persistent urticaria (necrotizing vasculitis), and there may be hypocomplementemia.

Transient eosinophilia is observed in urticaria from reactions to foods and drugs.

High levels of eosinophilia are present in the angioedema-urticaria-eosinophilia syndrome.

Special examinations: Screening for functional C1 esterase inhibitor.

Ultrasonography for early diagnosis of bowel involvement; if abdominal pain is present, this may indicate edema of the bowel.

Treatment

Try to prevent attacks by elimination of etiologic chemicals or drugs, e.g. aspirin and food additives, especially in chronic recurrent urticaria. Detection of the cause and its elimination is the most important step in the treatment but is rarely successful. The cause can be known from careful history taking rather than from laboratory investigations or skin testing.

Antihistamines are effective in controlling symptoms if given in the proper dose. H_1 blockers, e.g. hydroxyzine, ceterizine, levoceterizine; and if they fail, H_1 and H_2 blockers (e.g. doxepin).

Prednisolone is indicated for angioedema-urticaria-eosinophilia syndrome.

Danazol is indicated as long-term therapy for hereditary angioedema; whole plasma or C1 esterase inhibitor may be used in the acute attack.

Emergency cases: Emergency treatment should start with injection of adrenaline subcutaneously. Hydrocortisone intravenously should follow but not before adrenaline.

Topical soothing applications as calamine lotion can be used.

ERYTHEMA MULTIFORME
(Figs 7.2A to G)

Definition/Description

Erythema multiforme is a reaction of the skin to different causes as viral infections (commonly herpes simplex), bacterial, mycotic or parasitic infections, drugs, or systemic diseases (rheumatic fever, systemic lupus erythematosus, etc.). This reaction pattern of blood vessels in the dermis with secondary epidermal changes is exhibited clinically as characteristic erythematous iris-shaped papules and vesicobullous lesions typically involving the extremities (especially the palms and soles) and the mucous membranes. The characteristic lesions are also known as target lesions. The eruption begins rapidly with varying degrees of constitutional symptoms. It is distributed bilaterally and symmetrically in a centrifugal pattern. Stevens-Johnson syndrome is a severe bullous form of erythema multiforme. The mucous membranes are severely involved, and there are severe general constitutional symptoms.

Epidemiology/Etiology

Age and sex: Patients are usually 20 to 30 years old. 50% of cases are under the age of 20. Erythema multiforme is more frequent in males than in females.

Causes
Drugs: Sulfonamides, phenytoin, barbiturates, phenylbutazone, and penicillin.

Erythema multiforme
Dermatologic emergency

➤ Cause: Idiopathic in >50%
➤ Drugs: Sulfonamides, phenytoin, barbiturates, phenylbutazone, penicillin. Tracking for last 15 days
➤ Infection: herpes simplex, mycoplasma
➤ CF: Constitutional symptoms
➤ Mucosa-Ulcers over lip (99%), mouth (painful), cornea
➤ Skin-Macules, papules, vesicles, bullae, target lesions Bilateral, symmetrical over palms, soles, hands, feet, forearms, elbows, knees, penis System—Pulmonary manifestations
➤ Investigation: All attempts must be made to rule out occult viral, fungal, and bacterial infections
➤ DD: Childhood pemphigus
➤ Treatment: Remove/treat the cause if identified Symptomatic and supportive care Acyclovir to prevent recurrence due to herpes simplex Severely ill—prednisolone 50 to 80 mg daily in divided doses, quickly tapered

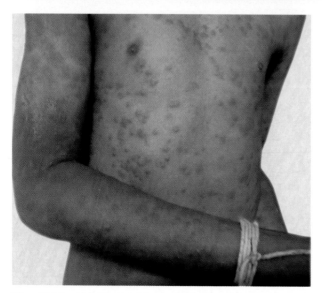

Fig. 7.2A: Erythmatous maculopapular rash following ampicillin. Few of them showing targetoid pattern in a child with EMF

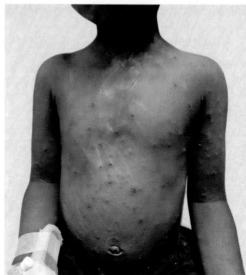

Fig. 7.2B: Erythematous maculopapular rash with target lesions in EMF

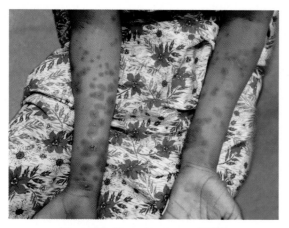

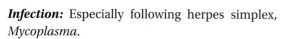

Fig. 7.2C: Target lesions of EMF

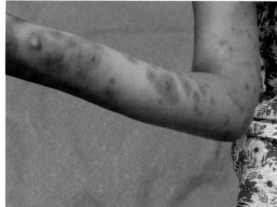

Fig. 7.2D: Erythematous papules, target lesions and bullous lesions in EMF

Infection: Especially following herpes simplex, *Mycoplasma*.

Idiopathic: In >50% of cases no cause can be detected.

Clinical Evaluation

The duration of lesions is several days; lesions develop over 10 days or more. Patients may have a history of prior episode of erythema multiforme. Skin lesions may be pruritic or painful. Mouth lesions are painful and tender. Constitutional symptoms may be present in the form of fever, weakness, and malaise.

Skin lesions: These consist of macules (48 hours) evolving to papules, 1 to 2 cm. Lesions may appear for 2 weeks.

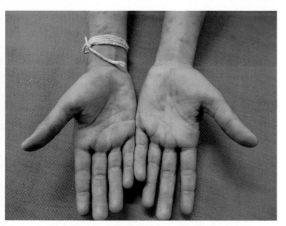

Fig. 7.2E: Involvement of palms with itchy erythematous plaques in a child with EMF

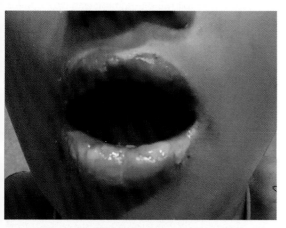

Fig. 7.2F: Mucosal involvement in EMF

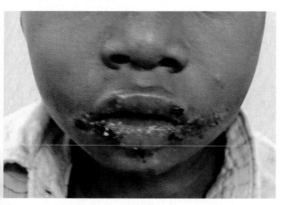

Fig. 7.2G: Hemorrhagic crusting of the lip in a child with EMF due to drug reaction

Vesicles and bullae (in the center of papule forming the so-called iris or target lesions).

Lesions are dull red. Iris or target lesions are typical (see above). Lesions may be localized to the hands or generalized. They are usually bilateral and often symmetrical. The sites of predilection include the dorsa of hands, palms, soles, forearms, feet, elbows and knees. The penis (50%) and vulva may be also involved.

Mucous membranes: Lesions may occur in the mouth and on the lips (99%).

Other organs: Pulmonary manifestations may be present. The eyes may be affected with corneal ulcers and anterior uveitis.

Investigations/Dermatopathology

Changes are observed in the epidermis and dermis. An inflammatory process is seen characterized by perivascular mononuclear infiltrate, and edema of the upper dermis; in lesions with bulla formation, there is eosinophilic necrosis of keratinocytes with subepidermal bulla formation.

All attempts must be made to rule out occult viral, fungal, and bacterial infections.

Treatment

Symptomatic. In severely ill patients, systemic corticosteroids are usually given (prednisolone 50 to 80 mg daily in divided doses, quickly tapered), but their effectiveness has not been established by controlled studies.

Control of herpes simplex using oral acyclovir may prevent development of recurrent erythema multiforme.

FIXED DRUG ERUPTION (Figs 7.3A to M)

Definition/Description

Fixed drug eruption is an adverse cutaneous reaction to an ingested drug, characterized by the formation of a solitary but, at times, multiple, plaque, bulla, or erosion. If the patient is

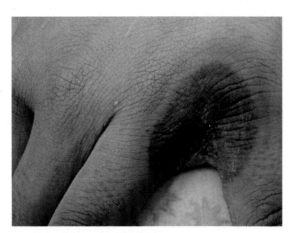

7.3A: Classical fixed-drug eruption with a rim of erythema surrounding the pigmentation

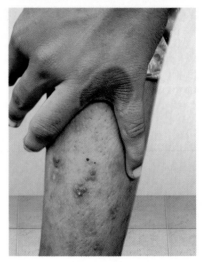

Fig. 7.3B: FDE following treatment with dapsone for treatment of lichen planus

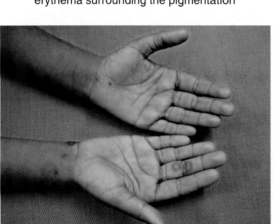

Fig. 7.3C: Adverse drug reaction started as FDE evolved into EMF in a child

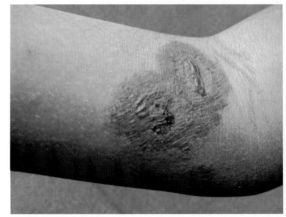

Fig. 7.3D: Bullous FDE that evolved into TEN. Note the acantholysis seen as erosion and new lesion close to the older one

rechallenged with the offending drug, the fixed-drug eruption occurs repeatedly at the identical skin site (i.e. fixed) within hours of ingestion.

Epidemiology/Etiology

The drugs most commonly reported to cause fixed drug eruption include barbiturates, phenacetin, pyrazolon derivatives (i.e. phenylbutazone), phe-nolphthalein, sulfonamides, and tetracyclines. The list of drugs causing fixed-drug eruption uncommonly includes many commonly used medications. The pathogenesis is unknown.

Clinical Evaluation

Fixed-drug eruption is usually asymptomatic but may be pruritic or burning and becomes

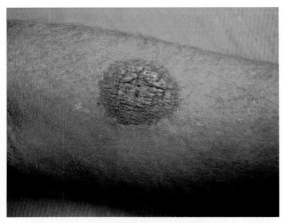

Fig. 7.3E: Bullous FDE that evolved into TEN

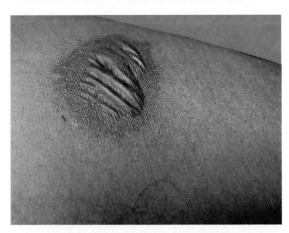

Fig. 7.3F: Classical bullous FDE

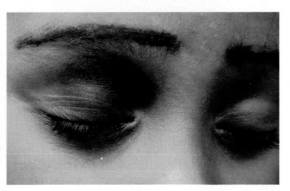

Fig. 7.3G: FDE of the eyelid with a risk of conjunctival involvement

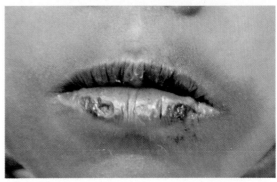

Fig. 7.3H: Itchy pigmented round patch following administration of cotrimoxazole—fixed-drug eruption

painful when eroded. Patients give a history of an identical lesion occurring at the identical location. Fixed-drug eruption may be associated with a headache for which the patient takes a barbiturate-containing analgesic, with constipation for which the patient takes a phenolphthalein-containing laxative, or with a cold for which the patient takes an over-the-counter medication containing a yellow dye. The offending "drug" in food dye-induced fixed-drug eruption may be difficult to identify, i.e. yellow dye in Galliano liqueur or phenolphthalein in maraschino cherries or quinine in tonic water.

Patients note a residual area of postinflammatory hyperpigmentation between episodes.

The characteristic early lesion is a sharply demarcated erythema, round or oval in shape, occurring within hours after ingestion of the offending drug. Most commonly, lesions are solitary but may be multiple. When multiple, the arrangement of the lesions is random. Size varies from a few millimeters up to 10 to 20 cm in diameter. Frequently, the edematous plaque evolves to become a bulla and then erosion. The color of the lesion is initially erythematous, then dusky-red to violaceous and, after healing, dark brown with vi-

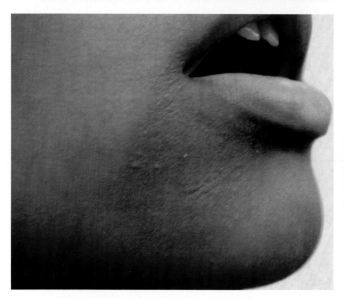

Fig. 7.3I: Pigmented patch in resolving FDE

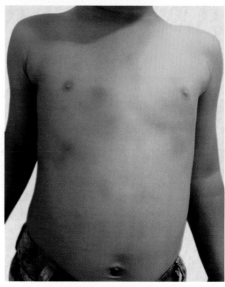

Fig. 7.3J: Multiple lesions of fixed-drug eruption following ibuprofen

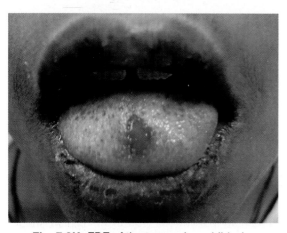

Fig. 7.3K: FDE of the tongue in a child who developed EMF

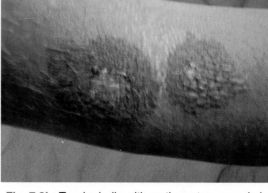

Fig. 7.3L: Tender bulla with erythematous margin in case of bullous FDE subsequently developed EMF

olet hue (postinflammatory hyperpigmentation). Eroded lesions, especially on genital or oral mucosa, are quite painful. The genital skin is the most commonly involved site. Fixed-drug eruption may also occur within the mouth or on the conjunctiva.

Investigations/Dermatopathology

The findings are similar to those of erythema multiforme, with dyskeratosis, basal vacuolization, dermal edema, and perivascular and interstitial lymphohistiocytic infiltrate, at times with eosinophils. Subepidermal vesicles and

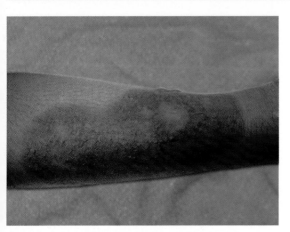

Fig. 7.3M: Large FDE with a potential risk to the development of toxic epidermal necrolysis

TOXIC EPIDERMAL NECROLYSIS
(Figs 7.4A and B)

Definition/Description

Toxic epidermal necrolysis (TEN) is a cutaneous drug-induced or idiopathic-reaction pattern characterized by tenderness and erythema of

---

Fixed-drug eruption

➤ Common agents: barbiturates, phenacetin, phenylbutazone, phenolphthalein, sulfonamides, tetracyclines
➤ *CF:* History identical lesion at the identical location Asymptomatic. May be pruritic or burning, painful sharply demarcated erythema, round, oval, patch solitary or multiple within hours become bulla and then painful erosion healing with pigmentation. Can involve mouth conjunctiva
➤ *Treatment:* Identify and withhold the offending drug Symptomatic: calamine lotion, betamethasone Oral sedative antihistamines Advice to avoid same or similar molecule

---

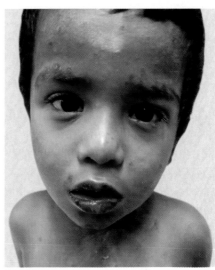

Fig. 7.4A: Conjunctival ingestion and hemorrhagic crusting over lips—caution sign towards toxic epidermal necrolysis

bullae with overlying epidermal necrosis may be also observed. Between outbreaks, the site of fixed-drug eruption shows marked pigmentary incontinence with melanin in macrophages in upper dermis.

Treatment
• Identify and withhold the offending drug.
• Symptomatic treatment of lesion(s) with topical calamine lotion or topical steroids (betamethasone). Oral sedative antihistamines are indicated when itching is severe.

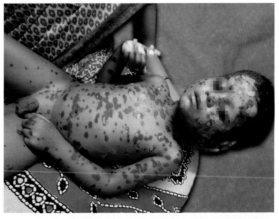

Fig. 7.4B: Full blown case of TEN shows positive Nikolsky's sign over apparently normal skin

skin and mucosa, followed by extensive cutaneous and mucosal exfoliation. It is potentially life threatening due to multisystem involvement. Patients become severely dehydrated and protein-depleted. They require intensive care and are best managed in a manner similar to burns patients.

Synonym: Lyell's syndrome.

Epidemiology/Etiology

Age and sex: Patients are usually adults more than 40 years old. The disease affects both sexes equally (some studies have reported a higher incidence in middle-aged and elderly women).

Causes

Drugs most commonly: Antibiotics, barbiturates, hydantoins, pyrazolone derivatives (phenylbutazone), sulfonamides, sulfones, and gold salts.

Other causes
Infections (viral, fungal, bacterial septicemia)
Vaccinations
Leukemia
Lymphoma
Graft-versus-host reaction
Idiopathic cases.

Clinical Evaluation

Ask about history of drug intake. TEN occurs within days of ingestion of the offending drug (when a drug is the cause); a newly added drug is most suspect. A prodrome occurs in the majority of patients and consists of mild-to-moderate skin tenderness, fever, malaise, headache, conjunctival burning or itching, myalgias, arthralgias, nausea and vomiting, and/or diarrhea. Skin symptoms are present in the form of marked tenderness of rash, pain, pruritus, and paresthesia. Patients are usually mentally alert, but are in distress due to severe pain. Acute renal failure and erosions in lower respiratory tract and gut may complicate the condition.

Toxic epidermal necrolysis
Lyell's syndrome Dermatological Emergency

➤ Causes: Drugs: antibiotics, barbiturates, hydantoins, phenylbutazone, sulfonamides, sulfones, gold salts
  Others: Infections, Vaccinations. Leukemia. Lymphoma. Graft-versus-host reaction. Idiopathic
➤ CF: Prodrome with morbilliform or erythema multiforme-like rash
  Pain, pruritus, paresthesia, bulla, marked tenderness of skin
  Positive nikolsky sign, epidermal sloughing, shedding of nail
  Acute renal failure, respiratory symptom, GIT complication
  Mucous membranes—severe involvement
➤ Investigation: Rule out infection as precipitating cause
  Treatment as thermal burn patient, with intensive care
  Use of corticosteroids – controversial (may arrest progression if given in the first 24 to 48 hours)
➤ Avoid re-exposure to offending allied group of drug

Skin findings: The prodromal rash is described as morbilliform or erythema multiforme-like. A tender erythema is initially observed. Small blisters then form, becoming irregularly confluent. The entire thickness of the epidermis becomes necrotic and shears off in large sheets, but large blisters only rarely form. Epidermal sloughing may be generalized, resulting in large denuded areas resembling a second-degree thermal burn. The idiopathic form is usually not preceded by rash but starts with erythema, which is rapidly followed by sloughing and denudation. The initial erythema affects the face and extremities, becoming confluent over a few hours or days. Denudation is most pronounced over pressure points. Scalp, palms, and soles may be less severely involved or spared, but nails may be shed. Nikolsky's sign is usually positive.

Mucous membranes are also severely affected; look for erythema and sloughing of lips, buccal mucosa, conjunctiva, genital, and anal skin.

The diagnosis is based on clinical findings and confirmed by biopsy.

Investigations/Dermatopathology

A biopsy will confirm the clinical diagnosis. Early findings include vacuolization/necrosis of basal keratinocytes and individual cell necrosis throughout the epidermis. Late lesions show necrosis of the entire epidermis with formation of subepidermal split above the basement membrane. Little or no inflammatory infiltrate is seen in the dermis.

Treatment

Treat as a thermal burn patient in a burn unit of a hospital. Silver sulfadiazine is extremely effective, but must be used with caution over large areas for fear of absorption and resultant neutropenia. The role of corticosteroids is controversial. There is general agreement that corticosteroids should not be used in TEN that has progressed to involve 20% or more of body surface. But, it is still unproven whether they may arrest the progression of TEN if given in the first 24 to 48 hours.

IV fluid replacement: Water, electrolytes, albumin, and plasma.

Debridement: Remove only frankly necrotic tissue.

Watch for signs of sepsis (fever, hypotension, and change in mental status).

Conjunctival care: Erythromycin ointment.

Frequent suctioning is needed in oropharyngeal involvement to prevent aspiration pneumonitis.

Avoid re-exposure to offending drug.

HENOCH-SCHÖNLEIN PURPURA (Fig. 7.5)

Definition/Description

This type affects children and young adults. Urticaria and purpura with multisystems involvement of kidneys, bowel, and joints characterize this type of purpura.

Epidemiology/Etiology

Damage to the walls of small blood vessels due to deposition of immune-complex substances. Cryoglobulins have been found rather than the immune complexes. An antigen associated with upper respiratory tract infection is suspected to be part of the usual cause of the immune response.

Clinical Evaluation

The manifestations usually begin with mild fever, sore throat, and upper respiratory tract infections, which may precede the skin rash. Macular rash appears first on the extensor surfaces of the limbs and buttocks, which becomes rapidly, urticarial and purpuric with central necrosis of the

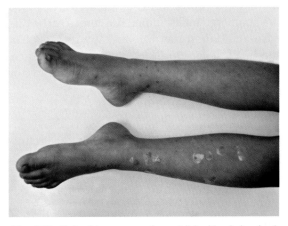

Fig. 7.5: Palpable purpura in a child with abdominal pain–Henoch Schönlein purpura

Henoch-Schönlein Purpura

➤ This affects children and young adults due to damage to the walls of small blood vessels due to deposition of immune-complex substances

➤ The manifestations usually begin with mild fever, sore throat, and upper respiratory tract infections which may precede the skin rash

➤ Renal, joint and bowel involvement are not uncommon

➤ Treatment of Henoch-Schönlein purpura is mostly supportive and includes ensuring adequate hydration and monitoring for abdominal and renal complications

➤ Nonsteroidal anti-inflammatory drugs (NSAIDs) may help joint pain and do not seem to worsen the purpura

➤ Clinicians often use corticosteroids to treat subcutaneous edema and nephritis

➤ Other treatment regimens have included IV or oral steroids with or without any of the following: azathioprine, cyclophosphamide, cyclosporine, dipyridamole, plasmapheresis, or high-dose IV immunoglobulin G (IVIG).

lesions. Renal involvement, which is focal nephritis. This is a serious manifestation of the disease. Bowel involvement leads to abdominal colic and hemorrhage. Polyarthritis and pain in the joints are another manifestations. The course of the disease is chronic. It may take weeks for regression of the skin lesions, but usually, there is recurrence. Renal and bowel manifestations may improve or may cause serious complications.

Investigations/Dermatopathology

Diagnosis of Henoch-Schönlein purpura is clinical and not based on laboratory evaluation. Routine laboratory test results are usually within reference ranges. Some laboratory studies help in excluding other diagnoses and in evaluating renal function, including urinalysis, CBC with platelet count and differential, BUN level, creatinine level, prothrombin time (PT), activated partial thromboplastin time (aPTT), and lipase level. Abdominal ultrasonography may be better than barium enema to diagnose intussusception, since Henoch-Schönlein purpura (HSP)–related intussusception is more often ileoileal instead of ileocolic as is typical in idiopathic intussusception.

Treatment

Treatment of Henoch-Schönlein purpura is mostly supportive and includes ensuring adequate hydration and monitoring for abdominal and renal complications. Nonsteroidal anti-inflammatory drugs (NSAIDs) may help joint pain and do not seem to worsen the purpura. However, NSAIDs should be used cautiously in patients with renal insufficiency. Clinicians often use corticosteroids to treat subcutaneous edema and nephritis, but few prospective placebo-controlled studies have demonstrated their effectiveness. Prednisone in a dose of 1 mg/kg/day for 2 weeks and then tapered over 2 more weeks has been shown to improve gastrointestinal and joint symptoms. Other treatment regimens have included IV or oral steroids with or without any of the following: azathioprine, cyclophosphamide, cyclosporine, dipyridamole, plasmapheresis, or high-dose IV immunoglobulin G (IVIG).

Papulosquamous Disorders

PSORIASIS (Figs 8.1A to K)

Definition/Description

Psoriasis, which affects 1.5 to 2.0% of the population in western countries, is a common, genetically determined, inflammatory and proliferative disease of the skin. The most characteristic lesions consist of chronic, sharply demarcated, dull-red (salmon pink) plaques surmounted by silvery white scales. The lesions tend to occur at sites of repeated minor trauma, particularly on the extensor prominences and in the scalp. The disease is variable in duration and extent and morphological variants are common.

Epidemiology/Etiology

One-third of patients are affected before 20 years of age. Females tend to develop psoriasis earlier than males. This earlier age of onset in females suggests a greater incidence in young females than young males. However, the incidence of psoriasis in adult men and women is usually reported to be about equal.

The evidence that psoriasis may be inherited is beyond doubt, and rests on population surveys, twin and other family analyses and HLA studies. Certain drugs (systemic corticosteroids, lithium, alcohol, chloroquine), sunlight, stress, and obesity are believed to cause exacerbation of

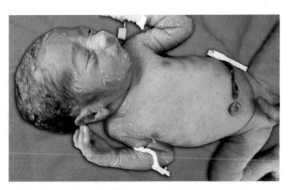

Fig. 8.1A: Congenital erythrodermic psoriasis in a 5-day-old neonate

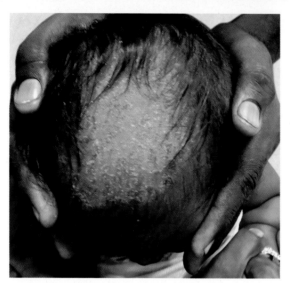

Fig. 8.1B: Classical erythematous plaque over scalp with silvery scale in congenital erythrodermic psoriasis

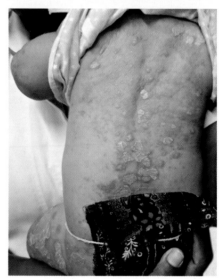

Fig. 8.1E: Classical erythematous plaque over the back with silvery scale in congenital erythrodermic psoriasis in an infant

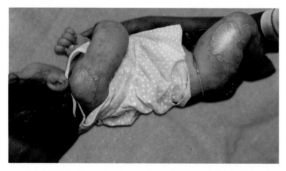

Fig. 8.1C: Classical erythematous plaque over limbs with silvery scale in congenital erythrodermic psoriasis in an infant

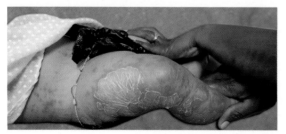

Fig. 8.1D: Classical erythematous plaque over the thigh with silvery scale in congenital erythrodermic psoriasis in an infant

pre-existing psoriasis. HIV infection must be considered in patients at risk.

Clinical Evaluation

Types

1. Salmon pink papules and plaques, sharply marginated with marked silvery-white scale. Removal of scale results in the appearance of miniscule blood droplets (Auspitz phenomenon).
2. Pustules (palmoplantar pustulosis).
3. Erythroderma (diffuse involvement without identifiable borders).

Pattern

1. Bilateral, rarely symmetrical. It most often spares exposed areas and favors elbows, knees, facial region, scalp, and intertriginous areas.
2. Disseminated small lesions without predilection of site (guttate psoriasis).

Hair and nails

1. Hair loss (alopecia) is not a common feature even with severe scalp involvement.

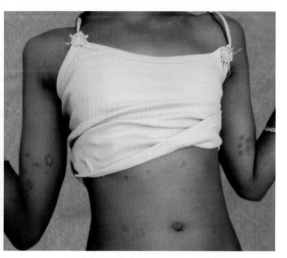

Fig. 8.1F: Early erythematous papules of psoriasis in a 9-year-old-girl

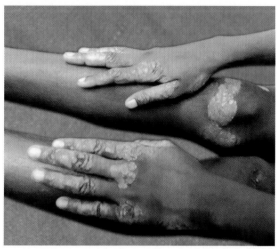

Fig. 8.1G: Classical erythematous plaque with silvery white scales over the extensor aspect of the knees and hands

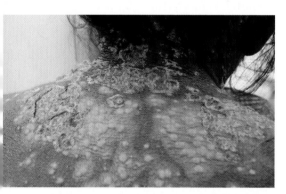

Fig. 8.1H: Superficial pustules coalescing to form lake of pus in a known case of psoriasis after sudden withdrawal of systemic steroid

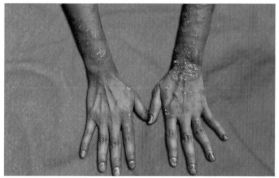

Fig. 8.1I: Pustular psoriasis in an older girl

2. Fingernails and toenails are frequently (25%) involved, especially with concomitant arthritis. Nail changes include:
   - Pitting (frequent but nonspecific)
   - Subungual hyperkeratosis
   - Onycholysis (also nonspecific)
   - Yellowish-brown spots under the nail plate—the "oil spot" (pathognomonic).

Arthritis: The incidence of psoriatic arthropathy (PA) is uncommon (3 to 4%) and more so in children.

Investigations/Dermatopathology

Dermatopathological changes in the epidermis and dermis are classical. There is alteration of the cell cycle (increased mitosis of keratinocytes, fibroblasts, and endothelial cells) with parakeratosis (clinically silvery scales), absence of granular cell layer, regular elongation of rete ridges with thickening of their lower portion (clubbing), elongation and edema of papillae (club-shaped) with dilated capillaries in the upper portion of the papillae (these are the earliest changes). Presence of

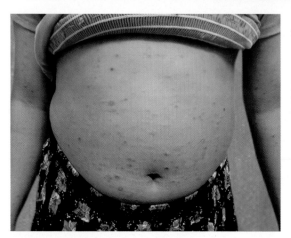

Fig. 8.1J: Erythematous scaly varioliform papules of Pityriasis lichenoides et varioliformis acuta mimicking guttate psoriasis

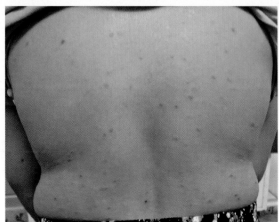

Fig. 8.1K: Erythematous scaly varioliform papules of Pityriasis lichenoides et varioliformis acuta mimicking guttate psoriasis

very small spongiform pustules in stratum malpighii (spongiform pustule of Kogoj – diagnostic), perivascular mononuclear cell infiltrate in upper dermis.

Sudden onset of psoriasis may be associated with HIV infection. Determination of HIV serostatus indicated in at-risk individuals.

Guttate psoriasis (guttate — Latin, "spots that resemble drops"), which is relatively rare (less than 2.0% of all psoriasis), is like an exanthem. A shower of lesions appears rather rapidly in young adults, often following streptococcal pharyngitis. Guttate psoriasis may, however, be chronic and unrelated to streptococcal infection.

Treatment

Topical mildly potent steroids like fluticasone/mometasone can be used for short intermittent courses. Systemic steroids are contraindicated. The resolution of lesions can be accelerated by UVB phototherapy or judicious exposure to sunlight. Penicillin or erythromycin are indicated if group A beta-hemolytic *Streptococcus* was isolated on throat culture

LICHEN PLANUS (Figs 8.2A to D)

Definition/Description

This acute or chronic inflammation of the skin and mucous membranes has characteristic flat-topped (Latin planus, "flat"), violaceous, shiny, pruritic papules on the skin, and milky-white papules in the mouth.

Epidemiology/Etiology

Most cases of lichen planus are seen in the 30–60 years age group, though children are commonly affected. Females are said to be affected rather more often than males, although an opposite ratio or equal sex incidence has been found in some studies.

The exact etiology is unknown, but severe emotional stress can precipitate an attack. Considerable evidence now exists that the underlying processes involved in the pathogenesis of lichen planus are immunologically mediated. It is also known that lichen planus can occur in families, and in these affected individuals an increased frequency of HLA-DR1, HLA-B7, HLA3 and HLA5 has been noted. Drugs may induce a lichen planus-like (lichenoid) eruption.

Psoriasis

➤ Genetically determined, inflammatory, proliferative disease of the skin and joint
➤ Exacerbated by drugs like beta blockers, lithium, alcohol, chloroquine, stress
➤ HIV infection must be considered in patients at risk
➤ *CF:* Sharply demarcated, salmon pink plaques surmounted by silvery white scales
  Auspitz sign, Koebners phenomenon
  Common types
  Guttate, plaque, pustular, erythrodermic, arthropathic
  Nail changes—pitting, subungual hyperkeratosis (SUHK), onycholysis, oil spot
➤ DD: Eczema
➤ Investigation: To rule out focal sepsis
➤ *Treatment*
  Topical – Emollient (liquid paraffin), mildly potent steroids short intermittent courses. Calcineurin inhibitors, calcipotrial
  Antibiotic in guttate psoriasis
  Systemic steroids are contraindicated
  UVB phototherapy or judicious exposure to sunlight
  Generalized pustular and erythrodermic psoriasis are dermatological emergencies
  Immunosuppresents used under professional guidance

Clinical Evaluation

Skin lesions: These consist of polygonal or oval, flat-topped, shiny papules, 1–10 mm in diameter, violaceous in color, with fine white lines (Wickham's striae) that are best seen with a hand lens after application of mineral oil. After disappearance of the lesions, a residual deep pigmentation is left and remains for several months.

Arrangement and distribution: The papules may remain discrete, or appear in groups, in lines, or in circles. Linear lesions often appear along scratch marks or in scars (Kobner's phenomenon). The papules may also coalesce into plaques. They are most commonly seen on the flexor aspects of the wrists, backs of the hands, lumbar region, glans penis (annular lesions), medial sides of the thighs, shins and ankles (thicker, hyperkeratotic lesions), eyelids, and scalp. Lichen planus actinicus occurs on sun-exposed sites. In guttate lichen planus, the papules are widely scattered and remain discrete.

Oral lesions: Oral lesions occur in 40 to 60% of patients and are seen on the buccal mucosa,

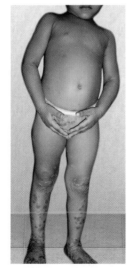

Fig. 8.2A: Itchy violaceous flat topped papules few coalescing to form plaques in a boy with lichen planus

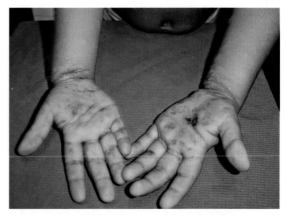

Fig. 8.2B: Lichen planus in a child

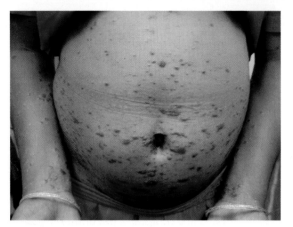

Fig. 8.2C: Genaralized lichen planus in a girl

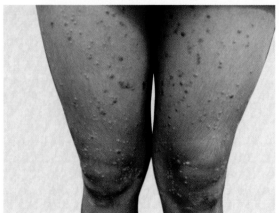

Fig. 8.2D: Generalized lichen planus over the thighs in the same girl as in Figure 8.2C

tongue and lips. The lesions consist of milky-white papules, with white lacework (white reticular streaks). Ulcerative lesions may also occur. Carcinoma may very rarely develop in mouth lesions. In 15% of the cases, the oral lesions are the only manifestation of lichen planus.

Hair and nails affection: Patches of atrophic cicatricial alopecia may occur on the scalp due to destruction of follicles by the inflammatory process.

Nail affection occurs in 10% of patients and presents as thinning and longitudinal ridging of the nail plate. Occasionally, an adhesion forms between the epidermis of the dorsal nail fold and the nail bed, causing partial destruction of the nail (pterygium unguis). Rarely, the nail is completely shed. There may be partial regrowth, or it may be permanently lost. The nails of the great toes are the ones most often affected in this way.

Squamous cell carcinoma may occur on lichen planus lesions of the oral mucosa (incidence 0.5%), on ulcers of the feet, and rarely on top of hypertrophic lichen planus.

Investigations/Dermatopathology

The epidermis shows orthokeratotic hyperkeratosis, focal hypergranulosis (this accounts clinically for Wickham's striae), irregular acanthosis, and irregular lengthening of rete ridges. There is also liquefaction degeneration of basal cell layer, with a band-like dermal infiltrate that closely approximates ("hugs") the basal layer that appears "wiped out." The infiltrate is formed mainly of lymphocytes and few histiocytes.

Treatment

General measures: Reassurance of the patient and avoidance of stress, sun and drugs causing lichenoid eruptions.

Lichen planus

➤ Etiology: Genetic, severe emotional stress, drugs like—beta-blockers, methyldopa, penicillamine, quinidine, quinine—lichenoid eruption.
➤ CF: Itchy, flat-topped, violaceous, shiny, polygonal papules . Wickham's striae, Koebner's phenomenon
➤ DD: Psoriasis
➤ Treatment: Reassurance avoidance of precipitating factor
  Topical—Fluorinated steroid creams and ointments, e.g., clobetasol propionate 0.05%.
  Systemic: Antihistamines (hydroxyzine hydrochloride).
  Steroids—acute generalized LP. Dapsone
  Oral lesions: Steroid in orabase

Topical preparations: Fluorinated steroid creams and ointments, e.g. clobetasol propionate 0.05%. 1% phenol in calamine lotion.

Tar preparations.

Systemic therapy: Tranquilizers and antihistamines may be used, e.g., hydroxyzine hydrochloride.

Systemic steroids, e.g. prednisolone 15–20 mg/day in short courses, are only indicated in severe cases, in acute generalized lichen planus, in ulcerative oral lesions, and when there is progressive nail destruction.

Oral photochemotherapy (PUVA) has also been advocated in the treatment of lichen planus with positive results. However, following a study that suggested that in some patients PUVA promotes carcinogenesis, the risk versus benefits of this form of therapy for use in a relatively benign disease must be seriously considered.

Oral lesions: Mouthwashes by triamcinolone; triamcinolone in a special base (Orabase) is sometimes helpful.

In very resistant oral lesions, cyclosporin A mouthwashes may be used.

Oral retinoids are also helpful for erosive lichen planus of the mouth.

Surgical excision of persistent ulcers has been recommended to guard against squamous cell carcinoma.

▌ PITYRIASIS ROSEA (Figs 8.3A to C)

Definition/Description

Pityriasis rosea is a benign, self-limited, exanthematous, maculopapular, red, scaling (Greek pityron, "bran") eruption that occurs largely on the trunk.

Epidemiology/Etiology

Pityriasis rosea affects 2% of dermatological outpatients. Most patients are 10 to 20 years old. The condition occurs more commonly in spring and autumn and one attack usually gives long-lasting immunity. For theses reasons an infectious (viral) etiology is strongly suspected though not yet proven.

Clinical Evaluation

Two forms of pityriasis rosea are described. The first form is of viral origin and is called primary pityyriasis rosea. The other form is the secondary pityriasis rosea, which is known to be a patterned reaction to:

- Seborrheic dermatitis
- Scabies
- Syphilis
- Sun exposure
- Drugs like barbiturates.

A "herald" patch precedes the exanthematous phase. The exanthematous phase develops over a period of 1 to 2 weeks. Pruritus may be present (mild or severe), or absent.

Skin lesions

Herald patch: (80% of patients) 2 to 5 cm, bright red with fine scaling. The herald patch usually occurs on the lower trunk or thighs, but may appear anywhere. In abortive pityriasis rosea, the condition is limited to the herald patch and does not proceed beyond.

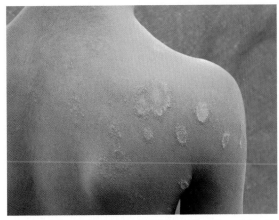

Fig. 8.3A: Herald patch of PR with sister patches

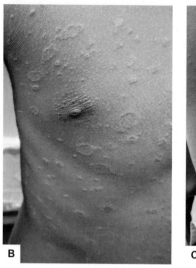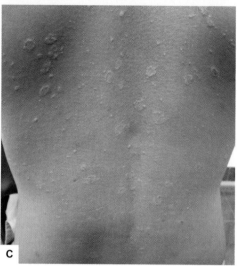

B   C

Figs 8.3B and C: Erythematous oval patches with peripheral collrette of scales of pityriasis rosea (trunk)

Pityriais rosea

➢ Features

Pityriasis rosea affects 2% of dermatological outpatients

Two forms of pityriasis rosea are described—primary and secondary. Herald patch is pathognomic

The lesions are oval, scattered, discrete and predominantly macular Fine, dull-pink or tawny, scaling, macules and papules with typical marginal collarette of thin scales

They are usually confined to trunk and proximal aspects of the limbs (vest and pants distribution)

But an inverted type of pityriasis rosea (on face and extremities)

➢ DD: Psoriasis and seborrheic dermatitis

Spontaneous remission usually takes place in 6 to 12 weeks or less

Topical mild steroids and oral antihistaminics are all that are required

Remnant hypopigmentation may last for some months

Exanthem: Fine, dull-pink or tawny, scaling, macules and papules with typical marginal collarette of thin scales. The lesions are oval, scattered, discrete and predominantly macular. They are usually confined to trunk and proximal aspects of the limbs (vest and pants distribution), but an inverted type of pityriasis rosea (on face and extremities) is also known. The long axes of the lesions follow the lines of cleavage in a "Christmas tree" distribution.

The condition has to be differentiated from

• Drug eruptions (e.g. captopril, gold, bismuth, barbiturates and clonidine).

• Secondary syphilis (serology is always positive).

• Guttate psoriasis (no marginal collarette).

• Erythema migrans with secondary lesions.

• Pityriasiform seborrheic dermatitis.

Investigations/Dermatopathology

Histopathology shows subacute and chronic dermatitis (spongiosis, exocytosis and dermal chronic inflammatory infiltrate). In addition, dyskeratotic eosinophilic keratinocytes and extravasated dermal RBCs may be seen.

Treatment

Spontaneous remission usually takes place in 6 to 12 weeks or less. If the eruption persists for over 8 weeks, a skin biopsy should be done to rule out parapsoriasis.

Symptomatic treatment like advice to avoid irritant woolen cloths, hot baths and soap. A mild corticosteroid cream and an oral antihistamine may help. Pruritus may be controlled by UVB treatment if this is begun in the first week of the eruption. The protocol is 5 consecutive exposures starting with 80% of the minimum erythema dose and increasing 20% each exposure.

Genetic Disorders

ICHTHYOSIS VULGARIS
(Figs 9.1A to E)

Definition/Description

Ichthyosis vulgaris (autosomal dominant ichthyosis) is a common disorder of keratinization, characterized by mild generalized scaliness clinically and reduction of the granular cell layer histologically. The disease is trivial and barely noticeable in most affected individuals but may be quite marked and disabling in a few patients.

Epidemiology/Etiology

The condition develops a few months after birth. It is inherited as an autosomal dominant disorder with equal incidence in males and females. It has been estimated that the gene occurs with a frequency of 1 in 500.

Histologically, the only abnormality detectable is a much-diminished granular cell layer. Ultrastructurally and biochemically, there is decreased content of a basic histidine-rich protein known as filaggrin, which is important in the orientation of the keratin tonofilaments. It is not known, however, how this abnormality leads to the increased binding between corneocytes and failure to desquamate, resulting in scaling. The rate of epidermal proliferation is normal. The scaling is regarded as a retention hyperkeratosis resulting from the increased adhesiveness of the stratum corneum.

Clinical Evaluation

There is generalized fine scaling over the entire skin surface, which tends to be worse in the winter time when humidity is low and may show improvement in the summer. The scaling spares the flexures (antecubital and popliteal fossae, and axillae) and is most noticeable over the extensor aspects of the limbs and trunk, being most conspicuous over the back, the lateral aspects of the upper arms, the anterolateral thighs, and

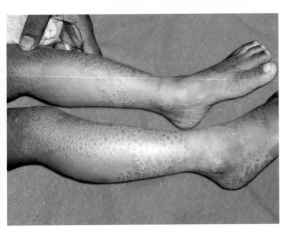

Fig. 9.1A: Ichthyosis vulgaris showing fish-like scales

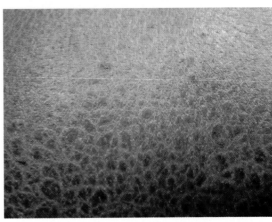

Fig. 9.1B: Close up view of fish-like scales in ichthyosis

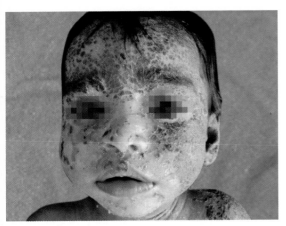

Fig. 9.1C: Involvement of face in a child with ichthyosis

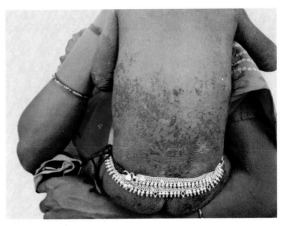

Fig. 9.1D: Large, polygonal and adherent (Fish-scale pattern) over back

particularly over the shins. The scales are large, polygonal and adherent (fish-scale pattern) on the extensor surfaces of the extremities, especially the shins; elsewhere they are small, powdery and skin-colored. Keratosis pilaris (follicular 'spines' due to plugging of follicular orifices by horny debris) may be seen over the outer aspects of the upper arms in a few subjects.

The condition is often mildly itchy and in the badly affected can cause some disablement because of the limitations imposed by the abnormal horny layer (splits and fissures occur, because of decreased elasticity).

Treatment

Emollients: Patients who have very severe scaling may apply topical keratolytic agents to some body sites, e.g. preparations containing urea in concentrations of 10–15% and salicylic acid in concentrations of 1–6%. The latter is particularly effective in encouraging desquamation but may not be used on large body areas for any length

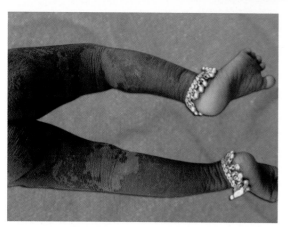

Fig. 9.1E: Large, polygonal and adherent (Fish-scale pattern) on the extensor surfaces of the extremities

---

Collodion baby

➢ AR ichthyosis with grotesque appearance encased in a thick collodion membrane
  CF: Fissures peeling of the membrane exposes red skin
  Ectropion, eclabium
  May turn normal, develop nonbullous ichthyosiform erythroderma or lamellar ichthyosis
➢ DD: Harlequin fetus
➢ Treatment: Special intensive care
  Maintain thermoregulation, hydration of the skin, correct of fluid, and electrolyte balance,
  Prevent infection
  Oral synthetic retinoids under supervision

Ichthyosis vulgaris

➢ AD disorder of keratinization
➢ CF: Generalized fine scaling over the entire skin surface sparing the flexures
  worse in winter with improvement in summer
  Keratosis pilaris, fissured feet
➢ DD: Other types of Ichthyosis
➢ *Treatment:* Emollients
  Moisturizers, keratolytics- urea 10–15% and salicylic acid in concentrations of 1–6%
  Oral retinoids (etretinate 0.5 mg/kg) may be used in very severe cases

---

Epidemiology/Etiology

The condition is known to occur once in 100,000 live births, more common in males, and in small-for-dates children. The disease is an autosomal recessive disorder with most of them ending with lámellar form of ichthyosis in about 60% of them.

Clinical Evaluation

At birth, the collodion baby is encased in a tight, shiny, moist membrane. As the membrane loses water by evaporation, fissures soon appear, the membrane contracts, and peeling of the membrane occurs, exposing the red skin beneath. There is accompanying ectropion and eclabium. The outcome is unpredictable. Some of them turn normal, while some develop non-bullous ichthyosiform erythroderma. Still others have chronic and severe lamellar ichthyosis.

Treatment

The mainstay is hydration of the skin, correction of fluid and electrolyte balance, and prevention of secondary bacterial and candidal infection. Special intensive care is to be administered in rooms of optimum temperature. Liberal application of

---

of time, as concentrations of more than 2% when applied to abnormal skin may cause salicylate intoxication (salicylism).

Oral retinoids (acitretin 0.5 mg/kg) may be used in severe cases.

COLLODION BABY (Figs 9.2A to D)

Definition/Description

This is a form of ichthyosis in which the newborn presents with a grotesque appearance as encased in a thick collodion membrane.

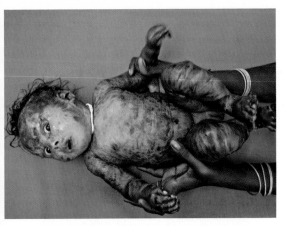

Fig. 9.2A: Infant covered with tight membrane with ectropion and eclabium in collodion baby

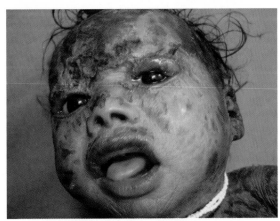

Fig. 9.2B: Collodion baby with ectropion

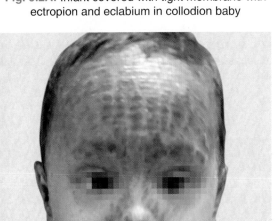

Fig. 9.2C: This 3-year-old was born as a collodion baby and treated with oral acitretin. Note the changes in the eyes

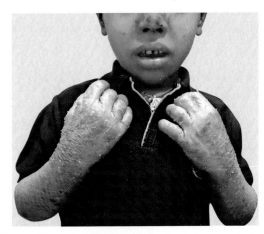

Fig. 9.2D: This 3-year-old was born as a collodion baby and treated with oral acitretin. Note the changes in the skin texture

emollients such as liquid paraffin but with minimum handling of the skin is essential. Early use of alphahydroxy acids, such as glycolic acid helps removal of the parched membrane. An antibiotic cover with ampicillin/cloxacillin remains essential. The genetic nature of the disease is to be explained to the parents and measures to prevent further offspring are to be emphasized. A visit 2 weeks after discharge from the newborn nursery is mandatory to evaluate specialized forms of therapy, such as oral synthetic retinoids.

ECTODERMAL DYSPLASIA (Figs 9.3A to D)

Definition/Description

Ectodermal dysplasia (ED) syndrome is a large, heterogeneous, nosologic group of inherited disorders that share primary defects in the development of 2 or more tissues derived from ectoderm. These tissues primarily are the skin, hair, nails, eccrine glands, and teeth. Defects in tissues derived from other embryologic layers are not uncommon.

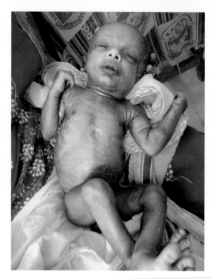

Fig. 9.3A: Infant with ichthyosis and ectodermal dysplasia

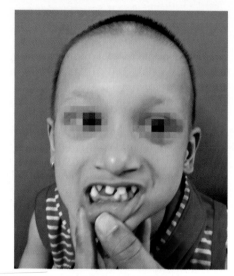

Fig. 9.3B: Conical teeth with diminished hair and absent sweating in a child with anhidrotic ectodermal dysplasia

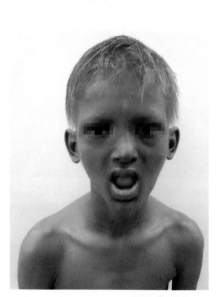

Fig. 9.3C: Ectodermal dysplasia with loss of teeth and loss of sweating

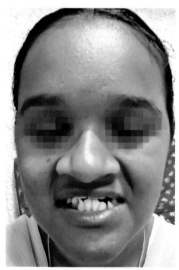

Fig. 9.3D: Hidrotic ectodermal dysplasia in an older girl

Epidemiology/Etiology

Current classification of ectodermal dysplasia (ED) is based on clinical features according to the presence or absence of (i) trichodysplasia, classified as subgroup 1, (ii) dental abnormalities, classified as subgroup 2, (iii) onychodysplasia, classified as subgroup 3, and (iv) dyshidrosis, classified as subgroup 4. The disorders are congenital, diffuse, and nonprogressive. More than 150 distinctive syndromes have been described with all possible modes of inheritance. ED results from the abnormal morphogenesis of cuticular or

Ectodermal dysplasia

➤ Ectodermal dysplasia (ED) syndrome is a large, heterogeneous, nosologic group of inherited disorders that share primary defects in the development of 2 or more tissues derived from ectoderm—the skin, hair, nails, eccrine glands, and teeth. Defects in tissues derived from other embryologic layers are not uncommon

➤ More than 150 distinctive syndromes have been described with all possible modes of inheritance

➤ The two best-defined syndromes within this group are:
  Hypohidrotic (anhidrotic) ED (also known as Christ-Siemens-Touraine syndrome) is the most common phenotype in this group and is usually inherited as an X-linked recessive trait
  Hidrotic ED (Clouston syndrome) is inherited in an autosomal dominant manner. The homozygous state may be lethal

➤ The care of affected patients depends on which ectodermal structures are involved

➤ For patients with anhidrosis/hypohidrosis, advise air conditioning for home, school, and work

➤ Encourage frequent consumption of cool liquids to maintain adequate hydration and thermoregulation. Finally, advise patients to wear cool clothing

➤ For patients with dental defects, advise early dental evaluation and intervention and encourage routine dental hygienen and dentures may be indicated as early as age 2 years. Patients with severe alopecia can wear wigs to improve their appearance

oral derivatives from embryonal ectoderm. The number of hair follicles, sweat glands, and sebaceous glands varies.

Clinical Evaluation

Clinical appearance depends on the anomalies of each syndrome. The two best-defined syndromes within this group are:

• Hypohidrotic (anhidrotic) ED (also known as Christ-Siemens-Touraine syndrome) is the most common phenotype in this group and is usually inherited as an X-linked recessive trait; autosomal recessive and autosomal dominant forms have been reported but are rare. It is characterized by several defects (e.g. hypohidrosis, anomalous dentition, onychodysplasia, hypotrichosis). Typical facies are characterized by frontal bossing; sunken cheeks; saddle nose; thick, everted lips; wrinkled, hyperpigmented skin around the eyes; and large, low-set ears. Because such characteristics are not obvious at birth, clinical clues for diagnosis in the neonatal period are extensive scaling of the skin and unexplained pyrexia. Dental manifestations include conical or pegged teeth, hypodontia or complete anodontia, and delayed eruption of permanent teeth. Most patients are fair-haired; therefore, little pigmentation in the hair shaft is observed microscopically and the medulla is often discontinuous. When medullation is present, a "bar code" (similar to those used for electronic control) appearance is common. The prevalence of atopic eczema is high. Other common signs are short stature, eye abnormalities, decreased tearing, and photophobia. Intelligence is normal

• Hidrotic ED (Clouston syndrome) is inherited in an autosomal dominant manner; the homozygous state may be lethal. Clinical features include nail dystrophy associated with hair defects and palmoplantar keratoderma. Nails are thickened and discolored; persistent paronychial infections are frequent. Scalp hair is very sparse, fine, and brittle. Eyebrows are thinned or absent. Patients have normal facies, no specific dental defect, and normal sweating.

Investigations/Dermatopathology

Structural hair-shaft abnormalities may result from aberrations in hair-bulb form and include longitudinal grooving, hair-shaft torsion, and cuticle ruffling. Hair bulbs may be distorted, bifid, and small. Eccrine sweat glands may be absent or sparse and rudimentary, particularly in those with hypohidrotic ED.

Treatment

The care of affected patients depends on which ectodermal structures are involved. For patients with anhidrosis/hypohidrosis, advise air conditioning for home, school, and work. Encourage frequent consumption of cool liquids to maintain adequate hydration and thermoregulation. Finally, advise patients to wear cool clothing. For patients with dental defects, advise early dental evaluation and intervention and encourage routine dental hygiene. Dentures may be indicated as early as age 2 years. Multiple replacements may be needed as the child grows, and dental implants may eventually be required. Patients with severe alopecia can wear wigs to improve their appearance. Patients with scalp erosions should be treated with topical and systemic antibiotics as needed. General scalp care may involve the use of weekly dilute bleach baths or acetic acid soaks to minimize bacterial colonization of the scalp. Application of special scalp dressings may be helpful. Artificial tears to prevent damage to the cornea in patients with reduced lacrimation help as do with saline sprays followed by the application of petrolatum to protect the nasal mucosa. Patients with ectodermal dysplasia with immunodeficiency should be monitored for infection and treated with therapeutic and/or prophylactic antibiotics when appropriate.

Bullous Disorders

EPIDERMOLYSIS BULLOSA (Figs 10.1A to D)

Definition/Description

These are a group of dermatoses characterized by easy bulla formation on mild mechanical pressure and, hence, the name mechanobullous disorders. The dreaded complications are bleeding, infection and scarring.

Epidemiology/Etiology

All forms of epidermolysis bullosa (EB) are genetic and most present at birth. There is no gender predilection. Most babies have impaired quality of life due to the psychological effects of easy blistering and scarring.

Clinical Evaluation

Several clinical types and subtypes have been described. Five of them need to be known.
1. EB of hands and feet (Weber-Cockayne). *Autosomal dominant.* The usual onset of recurrent blisters of hands and feet is in late childhood, with minimum scarring.
2. EB simplex. *Autosomal dominant.* Here the bullae are present at birth and present on the elbows and knees and other sites of friction, such as the dorsa of hands and feet.

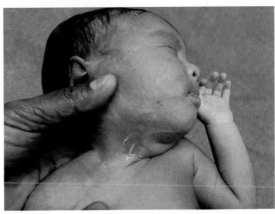

Fig. 10.1A: Erosion of skin following minimal mechanical pressure in a newborn with epidermolysis bullosa

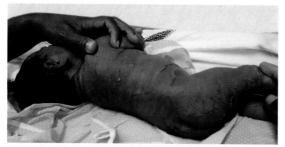

Fig. 10.1B: Erosions at the sites of mechanical trauma in a newborn with epidermolysis bullosa

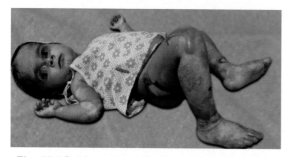

Fig. 10.1C: Hemorrhagic bullae, scarring in a child with junctional type of epidermolysis bullosa

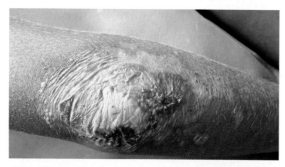

Fig. 10.1D: Dystrophic type of EB showing hemorrhagic bulla with scarring over the sites of trauma

Epidermolysis bullosa

➢ Inherited mechanobullous disorders mostly present at birth
➢ CF
EB of hands and feet—Weber-Cockayne blisters of hands and feet is in late childhood, with minimum scarring
EB simplex (AD)—At birth and present on the dorsa of hands and feet elbows and knees no milia minimal scarring
EB letalis (AR)—Generalized eruption on the skin and mucosae. Tracheal and bronchiolar involvement lead to respiratory distress. Infection and malnutrition lead to death
EB dystrophica (AR)—Onset at or shortly after birth Anemia Hemorrhagic bulla, milia scarring, webbed hands
EB dystrophica (AD)—Similar to recessive type less severe, associated with ichthyosis, keratosis pilaris, hyperhidrosis.
➢ Investment: Skin biopsy, Prenatal diagnosis
➢ Treatment: Essentially supportive
Sterile dressings and topical antibiotics (2% Mupirocin)
severe forms of EB—optimal care from the combined efforts of parents, pediatricians, dermatologists
➢ Genetic counseling

3. **EB letalis.** *Autosomal recessive.* In this form, generalized eruption of bullae occurs on the skin and mucosae. The oral mucosa is severely affected and interferes with feeding. Tracheal and bronchiolar involvement lead to respiratory distress. Infection and malnutrition lead to death.

4. **EB dystrophica.** Recessive. Blisters present at birth or shortly after birth. The disorder is characterized by bleeding into and from the blisters leading to severe anemia. The bleeding base heals with scarring which often entrap islands of epithelium, producing milia that appear as tiny, white cysts within scars. Scarring is often severe resulting in replacement of fingernails and pseudowebbing of all digits, leading to a club-like appearance.

5. **EB dystrophica.** Dominant. This form is less severe than its recessive counterpart but is often associated with ichthyosis, keratosis pilaris, and hyperhidrosis.

Treatment

Treatment of EB is essentially supportive. Sterile dressings and topical antibiotics (2% mupirocin) orm the mainstay of therapy. Cutaneous nfections unresponsive to topical antibiotics will need systemic antibiotics (cloxacillin). Nutritional support is essential in the form of soft flexible intragastric feeding in selected children. Attempts of intermittent esophageal dilatation may be fruitful. Apparently, the management of severe forms of EB demands optimal care from the combined efforts of parents, pediatricians, and dermatologists. Genetic counseling plays an important role.

STAPHYLOCOCCAL SCALDED SKIN SYNDROME (Figs 10.2A to C)

Definition/Description

Staphylococcal scalded skin syndrome (SSSS) is a toxin-mediated epidermolytic disease characterized by erythema and widespread detachment of the superficial layers of the epidermis, resembling the effects of scalding. It occurs mainly in newborns and infants under 2 years of age. Severity ranges from a localized form, bullous impetigo, to a generalized form with extensive epidermolysis and desquamation. Clinical spectrum of SSSS includes the following:

1. Bullous impetigo
2. Bullous impetigo with generalization
3. Scarlatiniform syndrome
4. Generalized scalded skin syndrome.

Synonyms: Pemphigus neonatorum, Ritter's disease.

Epidemiology/Etiology

Age: SSSS occurs mainly in infants and young children. Adults with immunosuppression or renal insufficiency are subject to SSSS.

Etiology: Staphylococcus aureus of phage group II, mostly type 71.

Clinical Evaluation

A low-grade fever may be present. The child is irritable.

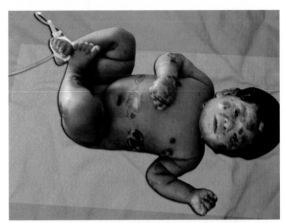

Fig. 10.2A: Multiple bullae and erosions of stahyloccal scalded skin syndrome

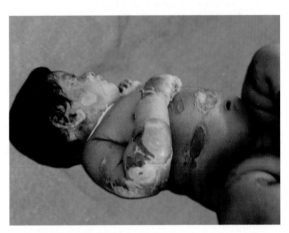

Fig. 10.2B: Multiple bullae and erosions of stahyloccal scalded skin syndrome over the front

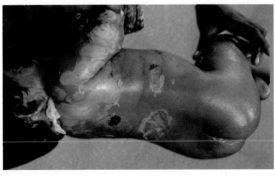

Fig. 10.2C: Multiple bullae and erosions of stahyloccal scalded skin syndrome over the back

Staphylococcal scalded skin syndrome

➤ Toxin-mediated epidermolytic disease, characterized by erythema and widespread detachment of the superficial layers of the epidermis, resembling the effects of scalding
➤ Clinical spectrum of SSSS includes:
  Bullous impetigo,
  Bullous impetigo with generalization
  Scarlatiniform syndrome
  Generalized scalded-skin syndrome-starts periorificially becoming more widespread, tender, ill-defined erythema erosions, positive Nikolsky's sign
➤ Mucous membranes: Usually uninvolved
➤ DD: TEN
➤ *Investigation:* Grams's stain-Gram-positive cocci only at colonized site like umbilical stump, not from erosion
➤ *Treatment:* Symptomatic treatment, topical—baths or compresses, antibiotic—mupirocin bacitracin, or silver sulfadiazine

Skin findings: Bullous impetigo: Lesions are often clustered in an intertriginous area and consist of intact flaccid, purulent bullae. Rupture of the bullae results in moist red and/or crusted erosive lesions.

Generalized SSSS: A very tender, ill-defined erythema occurs initially. With epidermolysis, the epidermis appears wrinkled. The unroofed epidermis forms erosions with red, moist base. Initially, lesions are present on the face (periorificially), neck, axillae, and groins, becoming more widespread in 24 to 48 hours. The initial erythema and later sloughing of the epidermis are most pronounced periorificially on the face, and in the flexural areas and pressure points on the neck, axillae, groins, antecubital area, and back.

Scarlatiniform syndrome: Presentation is like scarlet fever but without pharyngitis, tonsillitis, and strawberry tongue.

Nikolsky's sign (gentle lateral pressure causes shearing off of superficial epidermis) is positive.

Mucous membranes: They are usually uninvolved.

Investigations/Dermatopathology

Grams's stain

Bullous impetigo: Findings include pus in bullae and clumps of gram-positive cocci within PMNL.

Generalized SSSS: Gram-positive cocci are only observed at colonized site, not in areas of epidermolysis.

Bacterial culture

Bullous impetigo: Staph. aureus is isolated.

Generalized SSSS: Staph. aureus is only present in colonized site of infection, i.e. umbilical stump, conjunctiva, or external ear canal; culture of sloughing skin or bullae usually yields no pathogens.

Treatment

For a newborn, hospitalization and treatment with IV cloxacillin, 200 mg per kg body weight per day in divided every 4 hours, are preferable.

Hospitalize infants with extensive sloughing of skin or if parental compliance to treatment is questioned.

With reliable home care and mild involvement, cloxacillin, 30 to 50 mg per kg body weight per day, can be given orally.

Topical care includes baths or compresses, and mupirocin ointment, bacitracin, or silver sulfadiazine.

LINEAR IMMUNOGLOBULIN A (IgA) DERMATOSIS (Figs 10.3A and B)

Definition/Description

Linear immunoglobulin A (IgA) dermatosis (LAD) is an autoimmune subepidermal vesiculobullous

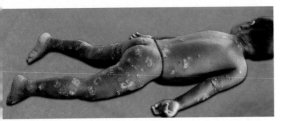

Fig. 10.3A: Tense bullae distribute over the extremities in linear IgA dermatosis

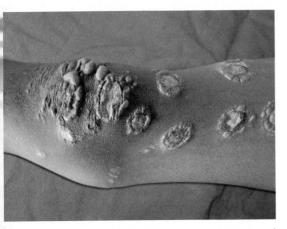

Fig. 10.3B: Tense vesicles in herpetiform pattern and few annular or polycyclic lesions

Linear immunoglobulin A (IgA) dermatosis

➤ Linear immunoglobulin A (IgA) dermatosis (LAD) is an autoimmune subepidermal vesiculobullous disease that may be idiopathic or drug-induced
➤ LAD is an autoimmune disease histopathologically characterized by the linear deposition of IgA at the basement membrane zone (BMZ)
➤ Some children have a prolonged period of prodromal itching or transient pruritus or burning before lesions appear
➤ The classic primary lesions of linear IgA dermatosis are clear and/or hemorrhagic round or oval vesicles or bullae on normal, erythematous, or urticarial skin
➤ Bullae may be discrete or arranged in a herpetiform pattern, often described as the cluster of jewels sign
➤ Histologically early urticarial papules or plaques reveal neutrophilic microabscesses in dermal papillae. Fully developed lesions reveal subepidermal blistering with a predominantly polymorphonuclear infiltrate, although mononuclear cells and eosinophils may be present. Direct immunofluorescence study of salt-split skin reveals IgA deposition
➤ Bullae do not need special care, as long they remain intact
➤ Infected lesions may be treated with topical mupirocin and sterile dressing changes twice daily
➤ Oral Dapsone is the drug of choice and the response of the condition to dapsone is almost confirmatory
➤ Oral steroids may be required in small doses for initial early resolution

disease that may be idiopathic or drug-induced. Children and adults are affected, with disease of the former historically referred to as chronic bullous dermatosis of childhood. The clinical presentation is heterogeneous and appears similar to other blistering diseases, such as bullous pemphigoid and dermatitis herpetiformis

Epidemiology/Etiology

Estimates have not been reported for LAD in children. The mean duration of idiopathic LAD of childhood is 3.9 years, ranging from 2.1–7.9 years. Remission occurs in most children within 2 years. Disease of adults is more protracted, with a mean duration of 5.6 years, lasting anywhere from 1–15 years. The remission rate in adults is less than

that in children (48%). The disease tends to wax and wane in severity. LAD is an autoimmune disease histopathologically characterized by the linear deposition of IgA at the basement membrane zone (BMZ). Antibody deposition leads to complement activation and neutrophil chemotaxis, which eventuates in loss of adhesion at the dermal-epidermal junction and in blister formation. Disease in children is immunologically identical to that of adults. The mechanism of loss of self-tolerance to target antigens is unknown. Within the dermal-epidermal junction, different antigenic target sites, including the lamina lucida, the sublamina densa, or both locations simultaneously, have been identified.

Clinical Evaluation

Some children have a prolonged period of prodromal itching or transient pruritus or burning before lesions appear. Patients with ocular manifestations may complain of pain, grittiness, or discharge. Bullae may be chronic, or lesions may appear acutely, as seen in drug-induced disease. Rash latency in vancomycin-induced cases of linear IgA dermatosis ranges from 1–13 days after the first dose. The classic primary lesions of linear IgA dermatosis are clear and/or hemorrhagic round or oval vesicles or bullae on normal, erythematous, or urticarial skin. Cutaneous manifestations may also include erythematous plaques, blanching macules and papules, or targetoid erythema multiforme–like lesions. Bullae may be discrete or arranged in a herpetiform pattern, often described as the cluster of jewels sign. Alternatively, vesicles and bullae may be seen at the edge of annular or polycyclic lesions, the appearance of which has been described as the string of beads sign. Lesions in children are typically localized to the lower abdomen and anogenital areas with frequent involvement of the perineum. Other sites of involvement include the feet, the hands, and the face, particularly the perioral area. Oral lesions include vesicles, ulcerations, erythematous patches, erosions, desquamative gingivitis, or erosive cheilitis, and they may precede skin lesions. Children and adults frequently complain of ocular symptoms, such as grittiness, burning, or discharge.

Investigations/Dermatopathology

Histologically early urticarial papules or plaques reveal neutrophils aligned along the BMZ accompanied by vacuolar change. Neutrophilic microabscesses may be seen in dermal papillae. Fully developed lesions reveal subepidermal blistering with a predominantly polymorphonuclear infiltrate, although mononuclear cells and eosinophils may be present. Direct immunofluorescence study of salt-split skin reveals IgA deposition on either the dermal side (blister floor) or the epidermal side (blister roof). Some patients demonstrate both linear IgA deposition and immunoglobulin G (IgG) deposition at the BMZ. Immunoglobulin M (IgM) deposition has rarely been reported. Serum should be obtained for indirect immunofluorescence studies. Approximately 50% of patients with LAD have detectable circulating antibody that binds to the BMZ.

Treatment

Bullae do not need special care, as long they remain intact. Ruptured lesions and erosions should be covered with sterile dressings. Infected lesions may be treated with topical mupirocin and sterile dressing changes twice daily. Patients with LAD can have changes, such as fine scarring, in the absence of ocular complaints. Therefore, most, if not all, patients once diagnosed should be see an ophthalmologist. Oral Dapsone is the drug of choice and the response of the condition to dapsone is almost confirmatory. Oral steroids may be required in small doses for initial early resolution.

Pigmentary Disorders

VITILIGO (Figs 11.1A to G)

The incidence of vitiligo is 1 to 8.8%. The age of onset varies widely from infancy to old age, with a peak incidence in the 10 to 30 years age group. The reported female predominance may be spurious, especially in India where vitiligo can be a considerable disfigurement and can affect eligibility for marriage, because vitiligo mimics leprosy.

The etiology is unknown. There is a positive family history in 30% of patients. An immune process is the most probable mechanism of destruction of melanocytes, as there are several autoimmune disorders, which occur with vitiligo: thyroiditis, adrenal insufficiency, and pernicious anemia, based on an autoimmune mechanism. An immune hypothesis would involve an aberration of immune surveillance that results in destruction of melanocytes. The primary event would be damage to melanocytes with the release of antigen and subsequent autoimmunization (probably in a genetically predisposed individual).

Clinical Evaluation

The white spots usually gradually appear and remain for life, with about 30% of patients reporting some limited spontaneous repigmentation. Rarely, vitiligo macules may be erythematous with a raised border and with itching. This "inflammatory" vitiligo has no special significance. Other findings in the history include premature graying of hair (<20 years of age), and history of halo nevi or alopecia areata. Skin lesions consist of white macules varying in size from 1 mm to large areas of the body. The typical color of these macules is "snow" white, but newly developing lesions may be "off-white" or even a light tan. Individual lesions are usually oval, forming geographic patterns; the borders may often be scalloped. There may be linear patterns or artifactual-type areas (as under a neck pendant); these represent the isomorphic or Koebner phenomenon. Pigmented or white hairs may be present in a vitiligo macule.

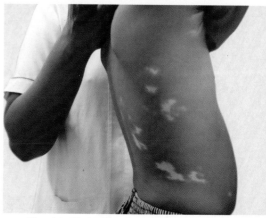

Fig. 11.1A: Isolated vitiligo areata in a 4-year-old

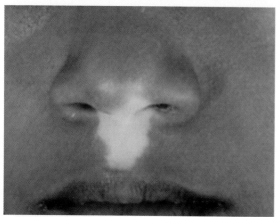

Fig. 11.1B: Vitiligo in segmental distribution

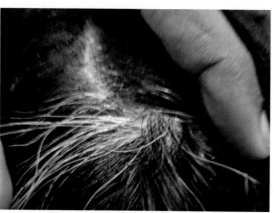

Fig. 11.1C: Depigmented asymptomatic patch with depigmented hairs in a child with vitiligo of the scalp

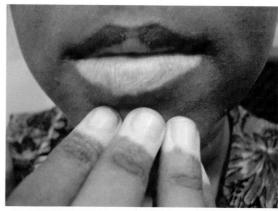

Fig. 11.1D: Depigmented asymptomatic patches with depigmented mucosa and skin over the finger tips in child—acrofacial vitiligo

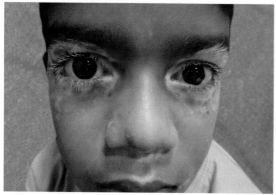

Fig. 11.1E: Periorificial vitiligo with depigmented hairs in a hypothyroid boy indicating poor prognosis

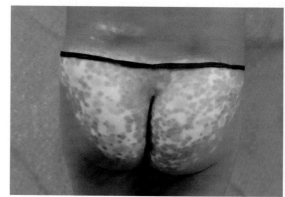

Fig. 11.1F: Contact depigmentation simulating vitiligo over the nappy area

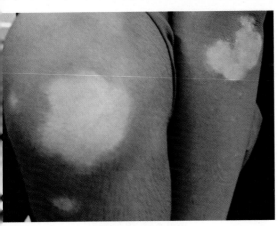

Fig. 11.1G: Depigmented asymptomatic patches of vitiligo vulgaris

---

Vitiligo

➤ *CF:* Round, oval, milky white, macules patches, scalloped margin
  Confetti macules, trichrome or quadrichrome
  Inflammatory border, leucotrichia in some
  Types: Localized (focal, segmental) or generalized
  Association: Iritis, thyroid disease, diabetes mellitus, pernicious anemia, addison's disease, polyendocrinopathy syndrome with mucocutaneous candidiasis
➤ DD: Post-inflammatory leukoderma
➤ Investigation: Wood's lamp to detect all the areas of vitiligo
➤ Treatment: Counseling
  Topical PUVA, steroid, calcineurin inhibitor
  Systemic PUVA (>10 yr of age). Avoid in photokoebnerization
  Hydroxy chloroquine in photokoebnerized cases

Distribution of lesions

Focal type: Isolated macules in one site.

Segmental: Unilateral, quasidermatomal.

Generalized: Multiple discrete macules, often strikingly symmetrical (in fact, mirror image) and at sites of repeated trauma, such as the bony prominences (malleoli, tip of the elbow, necklace area in females).

Mucous membranes: Lesions are rarely present in the mouth (gums).

Eye manifestations: Iritis occurs in 10%, but may not be symptomatic. Retinal changes consistent with healed chorioretinitis are seen in up to 30% of patients.

General examination: Search for thyroid disease (up to 30% in females), diabetes mellitus, pernicious anemia, Addison's disease, and polyendocrinopathy syndrome with mucocutaneous candidiasis.

Investigations/Dermatopathology

In the epidermis, melanocytes are absent in fully developed vitiligo macules, but at the margin of the white macules, melanocytes and a few lymphocytes may be present. There is also progressive destruction of melanocytes, possibly by cytolytic T cells.

Laboratory examination of blood

Serologic tests: ANA and other special tests for lupus erythematosus. Adrenal autoantibodies are found in 50% of patients who have Addison's disease.

Hematologic findings: These are normal, except in patients with pernicious anemia (obtain complete blood study including indices).

Blood chemistry: TSH (radioimmunoassay).
In Addison's disease: There may be a low fasting blood sugar, low sodium and high potassium, and an elevated BUN.
Fasting blood sugar should be done to exclude diabetes mellitus.

Wood's lamp examination: It is essential to examine patients with a light skin color with the Wood's lamp to detect all the areas of vitiligo.
Eye examination by an ophthalmologist is necessary before therapy.

Treatment

The treatment of vitiligo is best managed by a dermatologist who, depending on (i) concern about the disfigurement by the patient and (ii) the age of the patient, may choose topical PUVA photochemotherapy or oral PUVA photochemotherapy. In patients with extensive loss of normal pigmentation, "bleaching" the normal skin to make it totally white is a very satisfactory method of treatment. This is accomplished with topical preparations of monobenzylether of hydroquinone.

ALBINISM (Fig. 11.2)

Definition/Description

Albinism is a heritable disorder that affects skin, hair, and eyes. It principally involves the synthesis of melanin but also includes some alterations of the pathways of the CNS. Albinism can affect the eyes, ocular albinism (X-linked recessive), or the eyes and skin, oculocutaneous albinism. In oculocutaneous albinism, the disorder is autosomal recessive, with dilution of normal amounts of skin, hair, and melanin pigment; nystagmus and iris translucency are always present, and there is a reduction of visual acuity, sometimes severe enough to cause blindness.

Epidemiology/Etiology

The general incidence is 1:20,000. Albinism is present at birth. There is no special predilection in any one skin color. Hermansky-Pudlak syndrome (oculocutaneous albinism and a platelet disorder) is seen in Hispanics from Puerto Rico, in persons of Dutch origin, and in East Indians from Chennai.

Classification of oculocutaneous albinism: There are 10 types of oculocutaneous albinism, based on the following:
1. The level of tyrosinase in the plucked hair bulb (ty-positive and ty-negative)

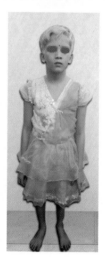

Fig. 11.2: Universal loss of pigment including the hair and iris since birth in a child with oculocutaneous albinism

2. Hair color (yellow, red, platinum), and
3. Associated problems, such as platelet abnormalities and ceroid storage disease (Hermansky-Pudlak syndrome) or defects in immunity (Chediak-Higashi syndrome).

Mode of inheritance is mostly autosomal recessive. Exceptions are the ocular forms that are X-linked recessive and those associated with deafness that are autosomal dominant.

Clinical Evaluation

Patients with albinism early in life avoid the sun, because of repeated sunburns, especially as toddlers. In Hermansky-Pudlak syndrome, there is also epistaxis, gingival bleeding, excessive bleeding after childbirth or tooth extraction, and fibrotic restrictive lung disease. There may be no family history of albinism in the autosomal recessive or X-linked recessive types. Albinos live an essentially normal life, except for problems with vision and, in lower latitudes, the development of skin cancers and dermatoheliosis. In some countries, there are volunteer groups, which assist albinos in various ways, especially in dealing with vision problems: obtaining driver's license, etc. Many albinos appear to be musicians and to be high achievers. The appearance of albinos is typical, with "poring" (eyes half closed, squinting) when in sunlight. Skin color is "snow"-white, fair, cream, or light tan. Hair is white (ty-neg), yellow cream, or light brown (ty-pos), and may be red, or platinum. The iris is translucent, with nystagmus.

Investigations/Dermatopathology

Light microscopy: Melanocytes are present in the skin and hair bulb in all types of albinism. The dopa reaction of the skin and hair is markedly reduced or absent in melanocytes of the skin and hair, depending on the type of albinism (ty-neg or ty-pos).

Electron microscopy: Melanosomes are present in melanocytes in all types of albinism, but depending on the type of albinism, there is a reduction of the melanization of melanosomes, with many being completely unmelanized (stage I) in ty-neg albinism. Melanosomes in the albino melanocytes are transferred in a normal manner to the keratinocytes.

Laboratory examination of blood: Morphologic, chemical, and functional defects of platelets are observed in Hermansky-Pudlak type of albinism.

Tyrosine hair bulb test (ty-neg and ty-pos): Hair bulbs are incubated in tyrosine solutions for 12 to 24 hours and develop new pigment formation from normal and ty-pos patients, but no new pigment formation is present in ty-neg albinism.

Albinism is an important disease to recognize early in life, in order to start prophylactic measures to prevent dermatoheliosis and skin cancer.

Treatment

Skin care: A lifetime program beginning in infancy is necessary and includes the following:

- Daily application of topical, potent, broad-spectrum sun-blocks, including lip sun-blocks

- Avoidance of sun exposure in the high solar intensity season during the hours of 1000 to 1500
- Yearly examination by a dermatologist to detect skin changes—skin cancers and dermatoheliosis
- Use of topical tretinoin for dermatoheliosis and for its possible prophylactic effect against sun-induced epithelial skin cancers.

Systemic beta-carotene (30 to 60 mg tid) imparts a more normal color to the skin and may possibly have some protective effect on the development of skin cancers.

PITYRIASIS ALBA (Fig. 11.3)

Clinical Evaluation

The individual lesion is a rounded, oval, or irregular plaque that is red, pink, or skin colored and has fine lamellar or branny scaling. Several patches usually are seen. Lesions usually range from 0.5 to 2 cm in diameter but may be larger, especially on the trunk. In children, the lesions often are confined to the face and are most common around the mouth, chin, and cheeks. In 20% of affected children, the neck, arms, and face are involved. Less commonly, the face is spared and scattered lesions are seen on the trunk and limbs.

Investigations/Dermatopathology

Histological changes are unimpressive. Acanthosis and mild spongiosis is seen, with moderate hyperkeratosis and patchy parakeratosis.

Pityriasis alba

See flow chart
Marker of Atopy
Spontaneous resolution
Rule out indeterminate Hansen
Emollient, TCI, mild steroid

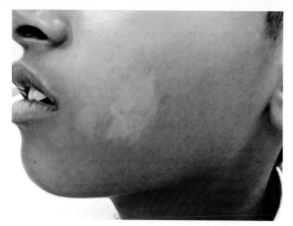

Fig. 11.3: Scaly ill-defined patch of pityriasis alba

Follicular plugging, spongiosis, and sebaceous gland atrophy may be seen. On electron microscopy, reduced numbers of active melanocytes and a decrease in number and size of melanosomes are seen in affected skin.

Treatment

Pityriasis alba resolves spontaneously and may not require treatment. Response to treatment often is disappointing. Treatment includes a simple emollient cream. For chronic lesions on the trunk, a mild tar paste may be helpful. Topical 1% hydrocortisone preparations may be helpful if mild inflammation is present. A variety of lotions, creams, and ointments, which contain hydrocarbons, oil, waxes, and long-chain fatty acids aid in retaining moisture in the skin, especially if applied immediately after bathing. A bland emollient may be used to reduce the scaling.

MONGOLIAN SPOT (Figs 11.4A and B)

Definition/Description

Mongolian spot refers to a macular blue-gray pigmentation usually on the sacral area of healthy infants. Mongolian spot is usually present at birth or appears within the first weeks of life. Mongolian spot typically disappears spontaneously within 4 years but can persist for life.

Epidemiology/Etiology

Mongolian spot is a congenital, developmental condition exclusively involving the skin. Mongolian spot results from entrapment of melanocytes in the dermis during their migration from the neural crest into the epidermis. This migration is regulated by exogenous peptide growth factors that work by the activation of tyrosine kinase receptors. It is postulated that accumulated metabolites, such as GM1 and heparan sulfate bind to this tyrosine kinase receptor and lead to severe neurologic manifestations and aberrant neural crest migration.

Clinical Evaluation

- Typically, it is a few centimeters in diameter, although much larger lesions also can occur. Lesions may be solitary or numerous
- Most commonly, Mongolian spot involves the lumbosacral area, but the buttocks, flanks, and shoulders may be affected in extensive lesions
- Generalized Mongolian spots involving large areas covering the entire posterior or anterior trunk and the extremities have been reported
- Several variants exist as follows:
    - Persistent Mongolian spots are larger, have sharper margins, and persist for many years
    - Aberrant Mongolian spots involve unusual sites such as the face or extremities
    - Persistent aberrant Mongolian spots also are referred to as macular-type blue nevi
    - Superimposed Mongolian spots, in which a darker Mongolian spot overlies a lighter one, have been described.
- Mongolian spots have been associated with cleft lip, spinal meningeal tumor, melanoma,

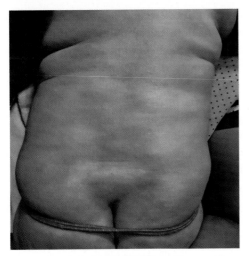

Fig. 11.4A: Typically located slate blue patches of Mongolian spots

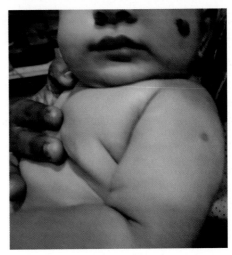

Fig. 11.4B: Aberrant Mongolian spot on the deltoid area—a sign of late resolution of lesions

Mongolian spot

➤ Mongolian spot refers to a macular blue-gray pigmentation usually on the sacral area of healthy infants, usually present at birth
➤ Mongolian spot results from entrapment of melanocytes in the dermis during their migration from the neural crest into the epidermis
➤ Typically, it is a few centimeters in diameter, although much larger lesions also can occur. Lesions may be solitary or numerous
➤ Mongolian spots have been associated with cleft lip, spinal meningeal tumor, melanoma, phakomatosis pigmentovascularis and with inborn errors of metabolism, the most common being Hurler syndrome. In such cases, the Mongolian spots are likely to persist rather than resolve
➤ Skin biopsy shows persistent melanocytes in the dermis
➤ Opaque cosmetics may be used as camouflage for Mongolian spots
➤ The value of lasers in Mongolian spot is uncertain
➤ Mongolian spots usually fade in the first year of life

phakomatosis pigmentovascularis and with inborn errors of metabolism, the most common being Hurler's syndrome. In such cases, the Mongolian spots are likely to persist rather than resolve.

Investigations/Dermatopathology

Skin biopsy shows persistent melanocytes in the dermis, some of them within macrophages (melanophages). In extensive Mongolian spots involving the back, radiographic studies are needed to rule out a spinal meningeal tumor or anomaly.

Treatment

Opaque cosmetics may be used as camouflage for Mongolian spots. The value of lasers in Mongolian spot is uncertain. Mongolian spots usually fade in the first year of life, but at times, they may persist indefinitely. Aberrant mongolian spots located in areas distal from the lumbosacral region may persist, unlike the typically located ones, which have a tendency to resolve.

CONGENITAL NEVOMELANOCYTIC NEVUS (Figs 11.5A and B)

Definition/Description

The congenital nevomelanocytic nevus (CNN), known commonly as the congenital hairy nevus, denotes a pigmented surface lesion present at birth.

Epidemiology/Etiology

CNN is present at birth or soon thereafter. The melanin pigment in the surface is apparent. Delay in appearance of surface pigmentation may occur from age 1 month to 2 years in the rare "tardier" type. A CNN larger than 9.9 cm in diameter occurs in 1 per 20,000 newborns and larger than 20 cm in diameter in 1 per 500,000 newborns. An equal prevalence exists in males and females. Autosomal dominant inheritance with incomplete penetrance or multifactorial determination occurs in families with small CNN.

Clinical Evaluation

The presence of a pigmented lesion is noted at birth or soon thereafter. Location and size of a congenital hairy nevus is variable. Small lesions appear more frequently than large lesions. About 5% of lesions are multiple. Coarse surface hairs develop in more than 50%. As described earlier the size varies from less than 1.5 cm to more than 20 cm in diameter. CNN may be located anywhere on the body, giving it names, such as 'stole nevus' (on the shoulder) and 'bathing trunk nevus' (over the whole trunk). They may be single or multiple and the borders may be sharp, regular, irregular, or may imperceptibly merge with the normal surrounding skin. The surface of CNN may or may not show hairs. Associated lesions include neurofibromata and leptomeningeal melanosis.

Investigations/Dermatopathology

CNN have nevomelanocytes in the epidermis as well-ordered clusters and in the dermis as sheets, nests, or cords. The presence of nevomelanocytes in the lower one-third of the reticular dermis is specific for CNN. Nevomelanocytes tend to occur in the skin appendages as well.

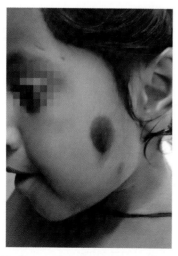

Fig. 11.5A: Congenital nevomelanocytic nevus over left cheek

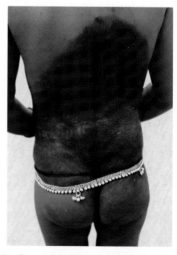

Fig. 11.5B: Congenital nevomelanocytic nevus over the back—bathing trunk nevus

Congenital nevomelanocytic nevus

> The congenital nevomelanocytic nevus (CNN), known commonly as the congenital hairy nevus, denotes a pigmented surface lesion present at birth

> Location and size of a congenital hairy nevus is variable. Small lesions appear more frequently than large lesions

> CNN have nevomelanocytes in the epidermis as well-ordered clusters and in the dermis as sheets, nests, or cords

> Two factors influence the treatment of congenital nevomelanocytic nevi, the potential for malignant change, and the cosmetic appearance

Treatment

Two factors influence the treatment of congenital nevomelanocytic nevi, the potential for malignant change and the cosmetic appearance.

Management and treatment of patients with CNN depends on size, location, and propensity for malignant transformation.

- Aesthetic considerations are important
- Surgical treatment of giant or large CNN is addressed at age 6 months
- Procedures used in surgical treatment include serial excision and reconstruction with skin grafting, tissue expansion, and local rotation flaps
- Adjunctive treatment options include chemical peels, dermabrasion, and laser surgeries
- Cultured epidermal autographs have been used successfully for select cases
- Removal of smaller lesions is delayed until adolescence. Management of small lesions includes close monitoring with photographic documentation.

ACANTHOSIS NIGRICANS (Figs 11.6A to D)

Definition/Description

Acanthosis nigricans (AN) is a diffuse velvety thickening and hyperpigmentation of the skin, chiefly in axillae and other body folds, the etiology of which may be related to factors of heredity, endocrine disorders, obesity, drug administration, and, in one form, malignancy.

Epidemiology/Etiology

Based on the etiology, AN may be classified as:

Type 1—Hereditary benign acanthosis nigricans where there is no associated endocrine disorder.

Type 2—Benign acanthosis nigricans which is often associated with various endocrine disorders, such as insulin-resistant diabetes mellitus, hyperandrogenic states, acromegaly/gigantism, Cushing's disease, glucocorticoid therapy, diethylstilbestrol/oral contraceptive, growth hormone therapy, hypogonadal syndromes with insulin resistance, Addison's disease, hypothyroidism.

Type 3—Pseudoacanthosis nigricans presenting as a complication of obesity. This is more commonly seen in patients with darker pigmentation. Obesity by itself is known to produce insulin resistance.

Type 4—Drug-induced acanthosis nigricans, examples of which include nicotinic acid in high dosage, stilbestrol in young males, oral or parenteral steroids.

Type 5—Malignant acanthosis nigricans-paraneoplastic syndrome usually associated with adenocarcinoma and less commonly with lymphoma.

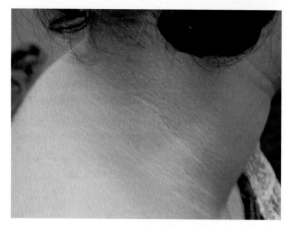

Fig. 11.6A: Early manifestation of acanthosis nigricans in a 6-year-old girl

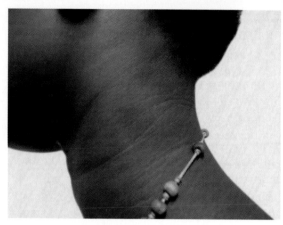

Fig. 11.6B: Acanthosis nigricans over the neck in a girl with wooly hair

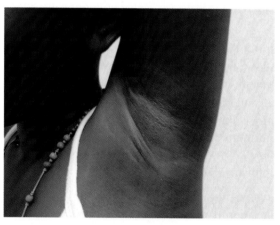

Fig. 11.6C: Acanthosis nigricans over the axilla a in girl with wooly hair

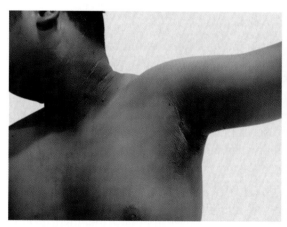

Fig. 11.6D: Pseudoacanthosis nigricans in an obese boy

Clinical Evaluation

The color of the lesions is dark due to accentuation of normal pigmentation.

The lesions appear verrucous but feel velvety on palpation.

Anatomical distribution of lesions includes most commonly, axillae, neck (back, sides), groins, anogenitalia, antecubital fossae, knuckles, submammary, and umbilicus.

In Type 5, mucous membranes and mucocutaneous junctions are commonly involved, with warty papillomatous thickenings periorbitally, and periorally.

General examination includes a search for underlying endocrine disorder in benign AN and a search for internal malignancy in malignant acanthosis nigricans.

Diagnosis is based on clinical findings. However AN has to be differentiated from confluent and reticulated papillomatosis (Gougerot-Carteaud syndrome—the finding of abundant pityrosporum orbiculare may support this diagnosis). Some

Acanthosis nigricans

➤ Acanthosis nigricans (AN) is a diffuse velvety thickening and hyperpigmentation of the skin, chiefly in axillae and other body folds

➤ Based on the etiology, AN may often be classified as five types

➤ The color of the lesions is dark due to accentuation of normal pigmentation

➤ The lesions appear verrucous but feel velvety on palpation

➤ Anatomical distribution of lesions includes most commonly, axillae, neck (back sides), groins, anogenitalia, antecubital fossae, knuckles, submammary, and umbilicus

➤ General examination includes a search for underlying endocrine disorder in benign AN and a search for internal malignancy in malignant acanthosis nigricans

➤ A combination of efforts, such as weight reduction and correction of endocrinopathy or insulin-resistance, if any, may be fruitful

➤ Topical keratolytics (0.025% tretinoin/3–6% salicylic acid) and chemical peeling with glycolic acid give temporary results

forms of verrucous epidermal nevi may show a clinical resemblance; but these are present from birth and are more localized.

Investigations/Dermatopathology

Dermatopathology shows hyperkeratosis, acanthosis, and papillomatosis; the epidermis is thrown into irregular folds, showing varying degrees of elongation of rete ridges with deeply pigmented basal layer. The epidermal changes may be caused by hypersecretion of pituitary peptide, or nonspecific growth-promoting effect of hyperinsulinemia.

Treatment

No single form of therapy is successful for AN. A combination of efforts, such as weight reduction and correction of endocrinopathy or insulin-resistance, if any, may be fruitful. Topical keratolytics (0.025% tretinoin/3—6% salicylic acid) and chemical peeling with glycolic acid give temporary results.

Nutritional Disorders

ZINC DEFICIENCY AND ACRODERMATITIS ENTEROPATHICA (Figs 12.1A to C)

Definition/Description

Acrodermatitis enteropathica is a genetic disorder of zinc absorption, presenting in infancy, characterized by a triad of acral dermatitis (face, hands, feet, anogenital), alopecia, and diarrhea; nearly identical clinical findings occur in older individuals with acquired zinc deficiency due either to dietary deficiency or failure of intestinal absorption.

Epidemiology/Etiology

Age
- Acrodermatitis enteropathica: in infants bottle-fed with bovine milk, days to few weeks. In breast-fed infants, soon after weaning
- Acquired zinc deficiency: older children.

Etiology
- Acrodermatitis enteropathica: autosomal recessive trait resulting in failure to absorb zinc
- Acquired zinc deficiency
- Secondary to reduced dietary intake of zinc
- Malabsorption (regional enteritis, following intestinal bypass surgery for obesity)
- Increased urinary loss (nephrotic syndrome)
- Prolonged parenteral nutrition without supplemental zinc.

Predisposition for acquired zinc deficiency: pregnancy, growing child, or adolescent.

Clinical Evaluation

Skin findings: The findings consist of patches and plaques of dry, scaly, eczematous skin, and perleche. The condition may evolve to vesiculobullous, pustular, erosive, and crusted lesions. Dermatitis occurs on palmar/digital creases, with fissures on fingertips, and paronychia. Annular

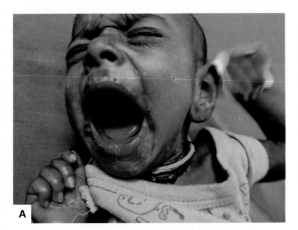
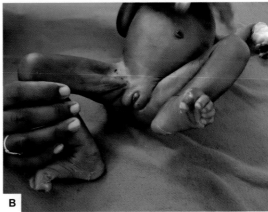

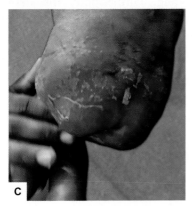

Figs 12.1A to C: Dry scaly eczematous erosive crusted peri oral perianal plaques, erythematous palms and soles and oral mucosa

Zinc deficiency and acrodermatitis enteropathica

➢ AR disorder of zinc absorption, of infancy, triad of acral dermatitis, alopecia, and diarrhea
➢ *CF:* Irritable, depressed mood, growth failure
    Skin: perioral, scalp, and anogenital area—dry, scaly, eczematous, vesiculobullous, pustular, erosive, crusted plaques,
    Annular lesions with collarette scaling
    Dermatitis on palmar/digital creases, fingertips,
    Impaired wound healing,
    Hair: Diffuse alopecia, premature graying of hair
    Nails: Paronychia, nail ridging, and loss of nails
    Mucous membranes: Oral: red, glossy tongue, superficial aphthous-like erosions, candidiasis, perlèche, photophobia
➢ DD: Leiners disease, Candidiasis
➢ Investigation: Anemia, low serum/plasma zinc levels, reduced urinary zinc excretion
➢ *Treatment:* Oral zinc in a dosage of 10 mg/kg of elemental zinc is as effective as parenteral administration continued for at least 6 months even up to adulthood

lesions also occur, with collarette scaling. The lesions often become secondarily infected with *Candida albicans* and *Staphylococcus aureus*. The lesions are initially pink, and later, brightly erythematous. They are initially confined to the face (particularly perioral), scalp, and anogenital area. Later, the hands and feet, flexural regions, and trunk become involved. There is impaired wound healing.

Hair: Diffuse alopecia, and graying of hair.

Nails: Paronychia, nail ridging, and loss of nails.

Mucous membranes: oral: red, glossy tongue, superficial aphthous-like erosions, oral candidiasis, and perlèche. Conjunctiva: photophobia.

General examination: patients are irritable, with depressed mood. Infants and children have growth failure.

Investigations/Dermatopathology

Complete blood count reveals anemia.

Chemistry: Serum/plasma zinc levels are low.

Urine: Urinary zinc excretion is reduced.

Dermatopathology: Intraepidermal clefts and blisters are observed with acantholysis.

Treatment

Dietary or IV supplementation with zinc salts with 2 to 3 times the recommended daily allowances restores normal zinc status in days to weeks. Oral zinc in a dosage of 10 mg/kg of elemental zinc is as effective as parenteral administration and needs to be continued for at least 6 months.

PHRYNODERMA (Figs 12.2A and B)

Definition/Description

Loewenthal first described the cutaneous findings associated with vitamin A deficiency (VAD) in 1933 when he described polygonal papules on the extensor surfaces of the extremities of patients who also had night blindness and xerophthalmia. The skin changes were later coined phrynoderma by Nicholls.

Epidemiology/Etiology

Internationally, at any one time, as many as 230 million children are at risk of clinical/subclinical VAD, and annually, more than 1 million deaths in children are associated with VAD. Females and males are affected equally. Avitaminosis A is most common in children aged 1–6 years, with the most severe, blinding complications affecting children aged 6 months to 3 years. The incidence is skewed toward children because infants born to mothers who are vitamin A deficient have small vitamin A stores at birth and, subsequently, get little from breastfeeding. Furthermore, the demands of rapid growth and susceptibility to infectious disease place an even greater demand on the meager body stores of vitamin A they do possess.

Clinical Evaluation

The most distinctive clinical features of VAD are present in the ocular system; however, numerous skin findings have also been reported. Generalized xerosis with fine wrinkles and scales may be present. Phrynoderma (follicular hyperkeratosis) is characterized by red-brown follicular papules that are approximately 2–6 mm in diameter, with

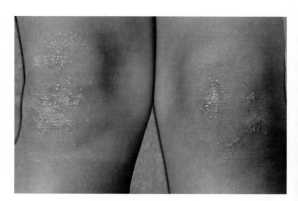

Fig. 12.2A: Horny foilicular papules of phrynoderma

Fig. 12.2B: Grouped horny keratotic papules bilaterally over knees in a child with phrynoderma

Phrynoderma

➢ Avitaminosis A is most common in children aged 1–6 years, with the most severe, binding complications affecting children aged 6 months to 3 years.
   The most distinctive clinical features of VAD are present in the ocular system
➢ Numerous skin findings have also been reported
➢ Generalized xerosis with fine wrinkles and scales may be present
➢ Phrynoderma (follicular hyperkeratosis) is characterized by red-brown follicular papules that are approximately 2–6 mm in diameter, with a central keratotic spinous plug
➢ The lesions are usually found clustered around the bony prominences of the elbows and the knees, although they may extend up the thighs and the arms
➢ Diagnosis is usually based on a high index of suspicion in children who are malnourished or in patients with predisposing factors for its development
➢ Medical care consists of oral administration of vitamin A 200,000 IU at presentation, the following day, and a third dose a week later is recommended
➢ Nutritional education is often
➢ Topical retinoic acid is of little value

a central keratotic spinous plug. These lesions are usually found clustered around the bony prominences of the elbows and the knees, although they may extend up the thighs and the arms.

Investigations/Dermatopathology

Diagnosis is usually based on a high index of suspicion in children who are malnourished or in patients with predisposing factors for its development. The biochemical definition of VAD is a plasma level of 35 micromol/dL or less. Several techniques are available, but high-pressure liquid chromatography is the most reliable. An important factor is that, with protein deficiency, serum vitamin A levels may be decreased despite good vitamin A intake and adequate vitamin A stores.

Treatment

Medical care consists of oral administration of vitamin A 200,000 IU at presentation, the following day, and a third dose a week later is recommended. Children younger than 1 year should receive one-half the standard dose, and infants younger than 6 months should receive a quarter of the standard dose. Common dietary sources of preformed vitamin A include liver, dairy products, and fish. Carrots are the major source of beta carotene. Other contributors of beta carotene are cantaloupe, broccoli, squash, peas, and spinach. Dietary modifications should include foods rich in vitamin A and periodic oral doses of vitamin A. Nutritional education is often incorporated into gardening projects and is provided at health centers in conjunction with the distribution of vitamin A supplements. Topical retinoic acid is of little value.

Index

Page numbers followed by *f* for figure and *t* for table, respectively.